# CHINESE PEDIATRIC MASSAGE THERAPY

*A Parent's & Practitioner's Guide to the Treatment and Prevention of Childhood Disease*

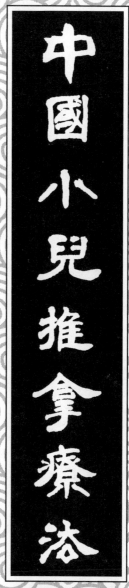

中國小兒推拿療法

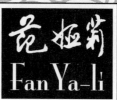

Fan Ya-li

BLUE POPPY PRESS

Published by:

**Blue Poppy Press**
**A Division of Blue Poppy Enterprises, Inc.**
**3450 Penrose Place, Suite 110**
**Boulder, CO 80301**
**Phone: (303) 447-8372**
**Fax: (303) 245-8362**

**First Edition May, 1994**
**Second Pringing March, 1999**

**ISBN 0-936185-54-6**
**LC # 94-74981**

COMP Designation: Original work

Printed on recycled paper at Johnson's Printing.
Cover design by Bob Schram at Bookends.

10, 9, 8, 7, 6, 5, 4, 3, 2

# Acknowledgements

First I would like to thank my husband, Dr. Nan Yun-sheng (南云生), for helping me with my English in writing this book and for all his support throughout this project.

I would also like to thank Dr. John R. Black of Nelson, New Zealand who patiently helped me revise my English drafts.

Thanks are also due Mrs. Kathyrn Liggett who first suggested and encouraged me to write this book.

And finally, I would like to thank Mr. Liu Bo ( 刘波) who drew the illustrations for this work.

# Preface

This book has been written in English by Dr. Fan Ya-li of the Shandong College of Traditional Chinese Medicine (TCM). Dr. Fan is a specialist in the treatment of disease with *tui na* or Chinese remedial massage. In particular, Dr. Fan specializes in the treatment of children's disease with *xiao er tui na* or Chinese infant massage. She has published several books in Chinese on Chinese infant massage as well as a dozen articles in TCM journals on the treatment of specific diseases with *xiao er tui na*. Dr. Fan has written this book in English in the hope that the unique benefits of Chinese infant massage may become more widely spread throughout the world.

Although references to Chinese infant massage within the Chinese medical literature go back to at least the *Nei Jing (The Inner Classic)*, the oldest and most authoritative Chinese medical classic, remedial infant massage came to the fore in Chinese medicine during the Ming dynasty (1368-1644 CE) when numerous books on this art were published. This art is based on many of the same theories as Chinese acupuncture and Chinese herbal medicine. For millennia the Chinese have believed that the internal functions of the body connect with the surface of the body via various pathways and channels and that one can effect internal functions and restore balance to the internal organs by manipulating certain points or areas on the surface of the body.

However, the Chinese also realized that infants are immature physiologically, anatomically, and energetically. They understood that the acupuncture points and channels operative in adults are not the same in children. Thus they developed a special repertoire of points and manipulations to restore balance to the infant's body distinct from adult acupuncture and massage. One of the characteristics of children is that they change very quickly. Therefore, they often do not need very strong medicine to initiate a return to health, and this is especially the case in most minor childhood diseases. For this reason, Chinese infant massage can often achieve quick results in the treatment of minor pediatric illnesses without side effects, drug complications, or the development of drug resistant strains. In particular, Chinese infant massage is an effective preventive and remedial therapy for children up to six years of age and, in general, is more effective the younger the child.

Chinese infant massage in China is typically administered on an out-patient basis in pediatric massage clinics in TCM hospitals. However, Dr. Fan, realizing that pediatric *tui na* can be learned and practiced by parents as well as professional physicians, has sought to publicize and teach this art to laypersons as well as Chinese doctors specializing in massage. In this book, she has presented simplified but nonetheless effective infant massage protocols for a number of common pediatric complaints. She has tried to make the differential diagnoses as simple and uncomplicated as possible. Although the more Chinese medical background one has the more one will get out of this book, the techniques Dr. Fan teaches in this book can be practiced safely and effectively even by TCM neophytes. Thus this book can be used as a textbook for teaching Chinese infant massage at both acupuncture/TCM colleges and massage schools, and it can be used as a clinical manual by acupuncturists and TCM practitioners, massage therapists, as well as parents and laypeople.

Laypersons using this book should first read the introductory material and the section on how to apply the most commonly used Chinese infant massage manipulations. They can then skip to the section on the disease in need of treatment. Because there are illustrations of the manipulation of each point in each protocol, beginners are not required to memorize the names, locations, indications, and methods of manipulation of a repertoire of points as in most Chinese professional pediatric *tui na* manuals. Students and professional practitioners, on the other hand, should read the entire book, should practice the main maneuvers, and familiarize themselves with the main points used. They should then keep this book on the shelf in their clinics ready for use.

The techniques in this book are specifically based on the Shandong school of pediatric *tui na*. There are several schools of pediatric *tui na* current in China today. Therefore, the manipulations and indications of some of the infant massage points described herein differ from those of other schools.

Bob Flaws
November 11, 1993

# Contents

## Book One
### The Basics of Chinese Pediatric Massage

## Book Two
### The Treatment of Common Pediatric Diseases

# Introduction

## Infant Massage, A Necessary Skill for All Parents

P arents' love for their children is great, lofty, sublime, and selfless. Since ancient times, countless legends, books, stories, and poems have praised this special parental love, for parents shower all their love on their children, frequently not even hesitating to sacrifice their own lives for their children.

### The parents' caress is the foundation of the child's health

As all parents know, being a parent is a joyful experience. A parents' love begins at the sound of their baby's first cry at birth. And when the child is sucking the mother's sweet milk and stroking her breasts with its small hands, a mother's love rises from her heart and flows into the baby's entire body with her milk. The response to this flow of love is the baby's serene look and dimple sweet smile. At such times, the mother may be immersed in the experience of boundless happiness and thus she may stroke the baby with her hands. Although this stroking may be done unconsciously, it plays a very important role in calming the baby's mind and promoting the circulation of their blood. Thus this stroking is very beneficial both psychologically and physically for young children.

Such stroking is a universal human instinct and a primitive form of massage. Modern Chinese infant massage therapy or *xiao er tui na* (小儿推拿) has gradually over the centuries developed out of this basic, primitive, instinctual stroking.

1

Therefore, when studying Chinese infant massage therapy, parents should first of all use their innate parental instinct and intuition. Especially mothers who do not or cannot breastfeed their babies should pay more attention to physically stroking their babies. It is my belief that more touching and stroking of infants can greatly enhance their physical and emotional health and well being.

## Love, but know how to love

Parents undoubtedly love their children. But the question is, do they know *how* to love their children? Some parents spoil their children by feeding them too much high protein foods, high energy, nourishing foods. They want to overfeed their children. But, as the saying goes, "You cannot build the body on one mouthful of food." Moreover, because a child's digestion is inherently immature and, therefore, weak, if they are overloaded, indigestion, lack of appetite, and even malnutrition may result. Such children will not be fat. On the contrary, for all the rich food they are given, they will still get thinner and thinner every day and their health will become poorer and poorer.

Some parents habitually worry about their children catching cold. Before the weather turns cold, they dress their children too heavily. Because of wearing such hot, heavy clothes, these children easily begin to sweat. To cool off they naturally take off these hot, heavy clothes (when their parents are not looking!) and then easily catch cold anyway. In addition, wearing heavy clothes can weaken a child's natural immune resistance. As it is said, "Hot house plants cannot stand wind and rain." Most people do not realize that frequently children's catching cold is caused by their parents' actions and not by external evils. Again the saying goes, "If you would make a baby healthy, keep them a little hungry and a little cold." Based on traditional Chinese medical theory, this seemingly odd statement does contain a kernel of truth.

Some parents have an excessive, blind faith in medicine and rely on it for their children's health. As soon as their children feel but a little uncomfortable, they rush them to the hospital to see the doctor with great apprehension. Such parents cannot rest at ease until their children have been prescribed and administered some modern medicine or been given an injection. The truth of the statement that "Whatever the medicine, it has some degree of toxicity" is never realized. Many modern medicines are quick acting but these also tend to have side effects and may weaken the child's natural resistance. Thus they may make the child ultimately more susceptible to disease in the future. Moreover, prolonged use of medicine can result in common germs developing sturdier strains resistant to medication. There are all too many children in China who have been frequent patients at hospitals since they were very young and have been repeat customers for intravenous drips, yet eventually even intravenous drips may not be able to achieve results in such resistant cases.

Therefore, parents must learn how to love their children wisely and how to help their children have healthy bodies. Traditional Chinese medical theory and practice, having developed over a period of not less than 2,500 years, can provide reasonable guidelines for the care and treatment of infants. Thus parents should dispel their unreasonable prejudices and beliefs and rather grasp the correct method of feeding and nursing. In addition, they can also try to understand some traditional Chinese medical knowledge and begin treating common pediatric diseases with *xiao er tui na*. Thus one's children will grow healthy under one's expert caress.

## Parents can be their child's doctor within the family

Many parents lack the confidence to care for their own children. They erroneously believe that medical theories are unfathomable and that disease may only be treated by professional doctors. Without doubt, the administration of medicine should be directed by a physician. However, those who have mastered the infant massage skills contained in this book no longer question the fact that parents can be doctors within the family.

Infant massage is, of course, not a universal cure, and seeing a doctor is sometimes necessary. However, many ailments can be treated effectively by parents with massage. In fact, children's diseases are, by and large, very simple. Only a few are serious and life-threatening. Most childhood diseases are common minor ailments that can be treated satisfactorily with massage. In such cases, massage treatment gets even better and certainly safer effects than modern medicines. Therefore, parents do not need to unduly rely on doctors for the treatment of childhood ailments.

For the treatment of many ailments, doctors who do not know the child's circumstances are not necessarily more effective than the parents. Nowadays, physicians tend to dispenses medicine exclusively, and many doctors habitually overprescribe these drugs which tend to be expensive and produce side effects. Although most doctors are aware of these side effects, they have, nonetheless, forgotten older, safer, more benign therapies such as Chinese infant massage. Thus frequent injections and hospitalization are prescribed, inflicting unnecessary pain and distress on children and their families.

It is my belief and experience that parents who have mastered basic Chinese infant massage skills are a good substitute for a cabinet full of medicine. Requiring nothing more than a pair of hands, this art can solve big problems. Using Chinese infant massage, children are spared the pain of injections and the side effects of drugs. Chinese infant massage categorically has no side effects. In addition, Chinese infant massage not only treats disease remedially but can also be used to prevent disease and promote even better health in the otherwise healthy. This is not something that can be done by modern doctors. As a clinician, I can say without hesitation that children treated frequently by Chinese infant massage are more healthy and less often sick than those treated by modern pharmaceutical. Thus I recommend the art of Chinese infant massage to parents everywhere and to practitioners worldwide who are looking for a safer, more humane, yet effective alternative to drug therapy for our *xiao peng you,* little friends.

# THE BASICS OF CHINESE PEDIATRIC MASSAGE

中國小兒推拿療法

BOOK ONE

# CHAPTER 1

# The Basic Theory of Chinese Pediatric Massage

The following is a brief introduction to the basic theories of Chinese pediatric *tui na*. As a part of Traditional Chinese Medicine or TCM, the more one knows and understands about TCM and its method of diagnoses and treatment, the better one will understand how to fashion and apply a pediatric *tui na* treatment. However, even those without previous knowledge of or professional training in TCM can successfully apply Chinese infant massage based on the principles discussed below.

## Suitable Ages for Treatment by Pediatric *Tui Na*

Chinese pediatric *tui na* is a special system of pediatric massage. It is specifically designed to prevent and treat pediatric disease and uses a special repertoire of points that are peculiar to children. Thus, Chinese pediatric *tui na* is only suitable for the treatment of children under 12 years of age. In particular, its effect is most pronounced in children under five. In general, one can say that the younger the age, the more effective is this method of treatment. For children over five, this treatment should be done in combination with appropriate adult *tui na* manipulations and adult points on the trunk, or it should be combined with medication.

## The General Requirements of Pediatric *Tui Na* Manipulations

Chinese infant massage manipulations are different from the general, simple, and casual movements of our daily lives. They are specific movements which require the development of special motor skills to do really well. And the level of skill in doing these manipulations is directly correlated to their clinical efficacy. Thus, in the course of practice, parents and professional practitioners should try to understand and gradually grasp these technically precise movements and manipulations. In that way, one can eventually learn to apply them skillfully not only in appearance but also in spirit.

In general, Chinese infant *tui na* manipulations should have the following characteristics: They should be persistent, forceful, even, and soft so as to be deep and thorough. Moreover, they manipulations should not be superficial or alternatingly heavy and light. Nor should they be too rapid or of too short duration.

## Characteristics of Points & Methods of Pediatric *Tui Na*

In addition to the points on the fourteen regular channels and extra-channel points of acupuncture, most pediatric *tui na* points are special points. These points are special because they are specific to the massage therapy of children and are only rarely used on adults. These special pediatric *tui na* points have three characteristics:

**1.** They are different from acupuncture points which only have a single, point-like form. Chinese pediatric massage points can be point-like, but they can also be line-like and area-like in shape. Thus there are three types of pediatric *tui na* points: point-like points, line-like points, and area-like points.

**2.** The special points of Chinese infant massage are mostly distributed on the hands and forearms. There are fewer on the head and face and quite a bit fewer yet on the chest, abdomen, back, and lower limbs.

**3.** The special points of Chinese infant massage are not connected by the channel and connecting vessel system as are the majority of points used in adult *tui na* or acupuncture/moxibustion. Thus the theory of their use is simpler to master.

As for the manipulations used in pediatric *tui na,* one uses different manipulations for points on different areas of the body. Generally speaking, when points on the torso and lower limbs are used for children, points located symmetrically are manipulated at the same time. Whereas, when special pediatric massage points are selected for stimulation on the arms or hands, their manipulation is often done on one side only. In ancient times, the doctor only stimulated points on a boy's left hand and a girl's right hand. Nowadays, this tradition is no longer observed, the left hand being used for the treatment of both sexes. If there is a cut or abrasion or any other problem of the skin or appendages which prevents treatment of the left hand, the right hand can be chosen instead.

## Duration of Treatment, Number of Repetitions, & Strength of Stimulation

The efficacy of a pediatric massage treatment are directly related to the quality of the massage manipulations. Using the same manipulations and points, some doctors attain good results while others attain no effect at all. In turn, the quality of a practitioner's manipulations depend upon the correctness of their physical shape and posture and on how correctly they have selected the points to be stimulated. In addition and even more importantly, one's results depend upon the skill and precision of the movements. This means flexibly understanding and applying the concepts of duration, numbers of repetitions, and strength of stimulation according to the child's specific conditions.

Generally speaking, for a one year old patient, when mild methods of manipulation, such as pushing, kneading, rubbing, and arc pushing, are used, they should be performed 200-300 times per point for the main points and 100-150 times per point for supplementary points. Based on this standard, children less than one year old should receive less repetitions and children more than one year old should receive proportionately more repetitions.

Chinese infant massage manipulations should be of appropriate force and softness as well as being even, deep, and thorough. In general, manipulations should be milder and slower for younger, thinner, weaker children and for those suffering from what TCM defines as vacuity patterns and chronic, debilitating diseases. For older, fatter, and stronger children and for those suffering from repletion patterns and diseases of short duration, one can use heavier, more forceful manipulations.

Typically, remedial pediatric massage treatments are performed once a day. However, this also depends upon the disease and the young patient's condition. For diseases accompanied by high or prominent fever, treatment may be repeated twice per day, while chronic diseases needing treatment over a long period of time can be treated in several courses. In that case, one course of treatment should last 7-10 days. One can either carry out treatment continuously without a break between courses, or one can rest for an interval of 1-2 days between each successive course.

## Indications & Contraindications of Pediatric Massage

In China, pediatric *tui na* is widely used. Almost all common pediatric diseases, including internal disorders, trauma, and diseases of the eyes, nose, mouth, and ears, can be treated effectively with pediatric tui na. In particular, Chinese infant massage especially and effectively treats pediatric digestive and respiratory disorders. Currently in China, the range of applicability of this unique art is being widened with the accumulation of practical, clinical experience. Based on the theories of TCM, new diseases are being treated with this ancient modality and pediatric *tui na* can also be used for the treatment of diseases which are otherwise not clearly understood. In such cases, quite miraculous effects can sometimes be gotten by Chinese infant massage.

## Other Important Points for Attention

**1.** Before performing massage, the parent's or practitioner's fingernails should be trimmed and rounded to an appropriate length. Their edges should be smooth and not jagged so as to avoid scratching the child. In addition, the therapist should warm their hands before laying them on the child. Otherwise the child will be startled and may begin to cry.

**2.** Since all infant massage manipulations are done directly on the child's skin, a suitable massage medium should be used in order to prevent chafing and to enhance the curative effects. The most commonly used medium in China today is talcum powder. In addition, one can use ginger juice, peppermint juice, or egg whites depending upon the condition of the patient and the disease being treated. Each of these media have their medicinal properties and functions according to TCM theory. When an appropriate medium is selected based on its TCM properties and functions, such a medium can increase the manipulations' efficacy.

**3.** One should be sure that the temperature in the treatment room is warm enough in winter and well ventilated in summer. In particular, one should ensure that there are no cold drafts which might chill the young patient.

**4.** The parents or practitioner should be careful and gentle with the child. They should avoid getting angry or rebuking the child during the therapy. On the contrary, the therapist, be they parent or professional, should direct all their love into the child's body.

**5.** Generally, the therapist should use their right hand for treatment while steadying and holding the child with their left. Both hands must work together cooperatively. The manipulations should be natural and smooth when changing from one point to another or when changing the position of the child. Dragging the child this way and that against their will should be avoided. In addition, the hand holding the child's limbs should not grasp too tightly, lest the child feel discomfort or pain and thus cry and interrupt the treatment.

## Common Pediatric *Tui Na* Points

Below are several diagrams (Fig. 1-4) showing the relative positions of the most commonly used pediatric *tui na* points.

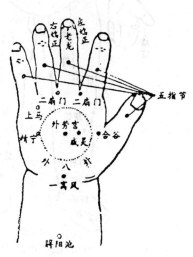

**Figure 1**

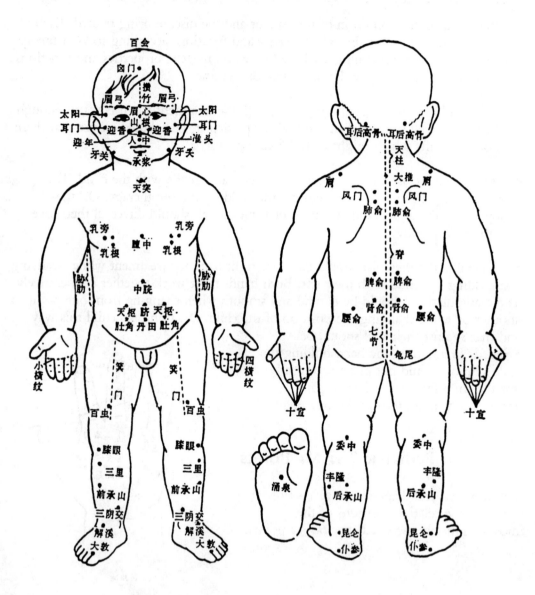

Figure 2                    Figure 3

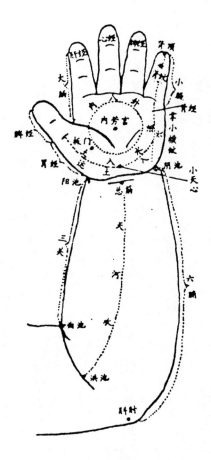

Figure 4

# Common Manipulations in Pediatric *Tui Na*

There are a number of basic Chinese infant massage manipulations which must first be learned before being able to put this safe and effective system of children's health care into practice. Below are descriptions of how to perform these common pediatric *tui na* manipulations.

## Straight pushing manipulation (*zhi tui fa*)

This method consists of pushing along a part of the body in a straight line. It is performed with either the therapist's thumb or the pads of their index and middle fingers. (Fig. 5) Throughout the movement, the fingertips must remain in close contact with the surface of the skin. The strength used should be steady and unfluctuating; and the movement should be done in a straight line and not obliquely. Typically, this method of manipulation is done at medium speed and is repeated continuously 100-200 times per minute.

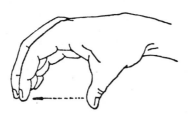 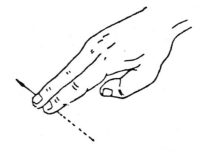

**Figure 5**

This is the most commonly used manipulation in pediatric *tui na*. It is suitable for treating all the so-called linear or line-like points requiring straight pushing from one point to another. Such "points" are, in fact, lines on the body even though they are called holes or points in Chinese similar to acupoints. It is a very easy manipulation to master.

## Pushing apart manipulation (*fen tui fa*)

This manipulation consists of pushing apart in opposite directions from the central point of a linelike point. One may use the fads of both thumbs or the index and middle fingers of both hands. The strength produced by the two hands should be even and equal. And, no matter whether pushing transversely or obliquely, the movement should be straight. The Chinese name for this method of manipulation can also be translated as separating pushing since one is as if separating or pulling apart a line on the surface of the body. (Fig. 6)

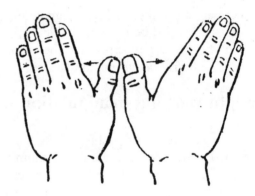

**Figure 6**

This manipulation is most often used on the forehead of the face, on the chest at the point between the nipples, on the abdomen under the ribs, and on the back. It should be done 100-200 times per minute.

# Kneading manipulation (*rou fa*)

This method of manipulation is accomplished by kneading a point or area in either a clockwise or counterclockwise circular motion. One can use either the finger tips, heel of the palm, or the thenar eminence below the thumb. In Chinese pediatric *tui na* there are several variations of this maneuver, each with their own names. For instance, there is finger kneading. This consists of kneading with one or two fingers. There is thumb kneading which consists of kneading with the tip of the thumb. There is heel of the palm kneading which is done by kneading with the bottom of the palm of the hand just below the wrist. And finally, there is thenar kneading. This is done by kneading with the thenar eminence just above the thumb. The thenar eminence is the large bulge of muscle above the thumb and below the wrist on the lateral, palmar side of the hand. (Fig. 7)

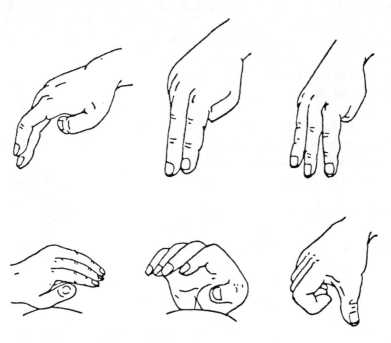

Figure 7

Kneading must be done with a soft, light touch, while its strength should be even and steady. The operating hand should remain fixed on the point being treated. It should not lose contact throughout the manipulation. In other words, there should not be any rubbing of the skin or slipping over the surface of the skin during this maneuver. Its frequency should be approximately 100-160 repetitions per minute.

This method of manipulation is suitable for almost every part of the body. Thumb and finger kneading are suitable for the treatment of every point-like point. Palm kneading is suitable for the belly. Thenar kneading is suitable for the limbs and face.

## Circular or round rubbing manipulation (*mo fa*)

This manipulation is accomplished by placing the palm of the hand or the palmar surfaces of the four fingers on an area of the child's body and then rubbing in a circle either clockwise or counterclockwise. Palmar circular rubbing consists of rubbing with the flat of the palm. Finger circular rubbing consists of rubbing with the palmar surfaces of the four fingers. (Fig. 8)

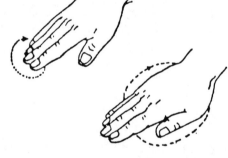

The frequency of this manipulation should be moderate and its performance should be even and steady. Its frequency is typically between 100-120 circles per minute.

This method is suitable for the treatment of the belly and is commonly used in digestive complaints.

**Figure 8**

## Pinching and pulling manipulation (*nie fa*)

This method is done by using either the finger tips of the thumbs, index, and middle fingers of both hands or the thumbs and lateral edges of the middle phalanges of index fingers of both hands. One grasps or pinches up the skin between these fingers at the point being massaged and then moves forward while rolling the skin with both hands upward. (Fig. 9)

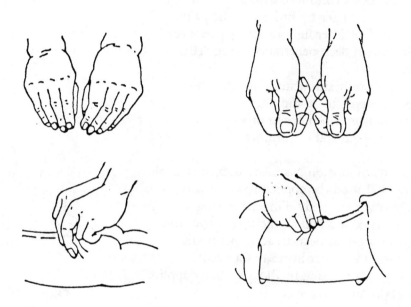

**Figure 9**

During this manipulation, the skin on the child's back should be fully exposed and the right amount of talcum powder or rice flour should be used as a medium in order to protect the child's skin from unwanted chafing. The strength of lifting should be moderate and the pinching should not be so tight as to cause pain. The rolling upward should be done straight upward without twisting or curving to the sides.

Clinically, this method is used for points along the child's spine. This is called spinal pinching maneuver. It is often used to strengthen the body in general and to prevent disease as well as to treat numerous diseases.

## Pressing manipulation (*an fa*)

Pressing as a *tui na* manipulation or method consists of pressing a particular point or area of the body continuously either with the therapist's finger tip or heel of the palm. It may involve either light or heavy pressure and shallow or deep penetration. (Fig. 10)

This is a strongly stimulating manipulation. It is often used after kneading, in which case one presses 3-5 times in order to relieve local pain and discomfort.

Pressing manipulation has many uses in clinical practice, and it can be applied to essentially all points over the body. Finger pressing method can be used on all the points over the body, and it can achieve an acupuncture-like effect using the finger instead of a needle, whereas, palm pressing method is chiefly applied to the abdominal area.

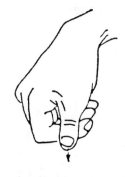
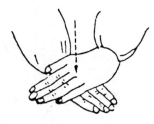

**Figure 10**

## Nipping manipulation (*qia fa*)

This method of stimulating a point by pinching it forcefully with the fingernails is called nipping manipulation. (Fig. 11)

When applying nipping manipulation, the pressure should be increased gradually. Attention must be paid to avoiding damaging the skin. When using nipping method, one should repeat this maneuver 3-5

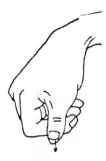

**Figure 11**

times forcefully per treatment. It is also a strongly stimulating manipulation. It is often used along with kneading. In this case, one first nips forcefully and then kneads in order to relieve local pain and discomfort. This method is suitable for all points over the body.

## Arc pushing manipulation (*yun fa*)

This method is accomplished by lightly pushing with the therapist's fingertips or surface of their thumb in an arc or circle around the place to be manipulated. Therefore, this maneuver is called arc pushing. (Fig. 12)

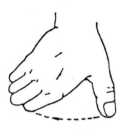

**Figure 12**

The strength used in doing this manipulation should be light and the speed of pushing should be slow. The rubbing should be soft and gentle, and the arc described by the moving thumb should be semi-circular or circular. The strength used for this manipulation should be much lighter than that used with round rubbing, and its frequency should be 80-100 times per minute. In particular, this method of manipulation is used for stimulating the points of the palm.

## Grasping manipulation (*na fa*)

This manipulation is performed by slowly lifting and squeezing a point or area of the body with the therapist's thumb and index and middle fingers. It may also be done using all five fingers on each hand. One grasps, lifts, and then releases. Thus this manipulation is called grasping. (Fig. 13)

This another strongly stimulating manipulation. It is mainly applied to points on the neck and shoulders, the sides of the abdomen, and the extremities. It should be

21

done last of all the maneuvers in a treatment session since its stimulation is strong and after applying this maneuver, for instance to the abdomen, the child may not let the therapist perform subsequent manipulations. Grasping is typically done 3-5 times per treatment.

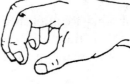

**Figure 13**

# THE TREATMENT OF COMMON PEDIATRIC DISEASES

中國小兒推拿療法

BOOK TWO

# Treatment Based on Pattern Discrimination

The foundation and hallmark of TCM as a style of medicine is the belief that each patient should receive individualized treatment. Modern Western medicine is primarily disease oriented. Every patient with the same disease typically receives the same or similar medicine or treatment. In TCM, however, the practitioner emphasizes the individual pattern of the patient over and above their disease diagnosis. Thus two patients with the same disease will receive different treatments if their overall patterns are different, while two patients with different diseases will receive the same treatment if their overall pattern is the same.

Thus the reader will see in the chapters that follow on the treatment of specific diseases that treatments for a single disease vary depending upon the pattern of the patient with that disease. Therefore, the parent or practitioner is guided in making a differential diagnosis before picking their treatment methods. In each disease, there are typically a few commonly encountered patterns. We have endeavored to keep these pattern discriminations as simple as possible. The better one can differentiate their young patient's pattern the more likely it is that the treatment chosen will achieve its desired effect.

CHAPTER
1

# Diarrhea

Diarrhea is a common pediatric complaint involving the digestive tract. In general, it is a form of indigestion. In particular, it refers to increased frequency in bowel movements with thin or even watery stool. Diarrhea can occur in any season, but in China it is most commonly seen in the summer and fall. If it is not given timely treatment and is allowed to continue for some time, it can affect the child's nutrition and thus their growth. Serious cases of diarrhea can cause such critical conditions as dehydration and acidosis, and may even endanger life. Thus diarrhea in children should be treated promptly and comprehensively.

Chinese pediatric massage is a highly effective treatment for children's diarrhea. Many children with diarrhea are not responsive to medication but are highly responsive to massage. Providing that the pattern diagnosis, point selection, and manipulation are correct, most cases of pediatric diarrhea will recover within three days.

## Patterns & Their Treatment

### Cold damp pattern (*han shi xing*)

**Disease causes:** This type of pediatric diarrhea is caused by evil cold and dampness affecting the spleen and stomach. Evil cold can be due to excessive eating of raw fruits and raw vegetables, chilled drinks, such as chilled fruit juices, and frozen foods, such as ice cream. It may also be due to exposure to climatic cold. Dampness may be due to excessive eating of damp foods, such as wheat products, dairy products, and many fruits and fruit juices, such as orange juice. Any food which is sweet tasting has the ability to generate dampness. The sweeter the food is, the more likely it is that it may generate evil dampness. In addition, living in a damp climate may also cause evil dampness resulting in diarrhea. Thus in China, cold damp pattern diarrhea is frequently seen in the late fall, winter, and early spring.

**Main signs & symptoms:** Loose stools, possibly with foam, or watery stools, light colored stools without offensive odor, rumbling intestines, abdominal pain, a pale face, no thirst, cold extremities, and frequent, excessive urination which is lighter than normal in color

**Treatment principles:** Warm yang, disperse cold, and stop diarrhea

**Treatment methods: 1.** Slightly stretch out the child's thumb and rub the line on the lateral palmar edge of the thumb, pushing in one direction only from the tip to the base of the thumb 100-500 times. (Fig. 14) This area encompasses two points called *Pi Jing* (Spleen Channel) in Chinese. This maneuver is technically referred to as supplementing the Spleen Channel. Stimulation of this point in this manner supplements the spleen.

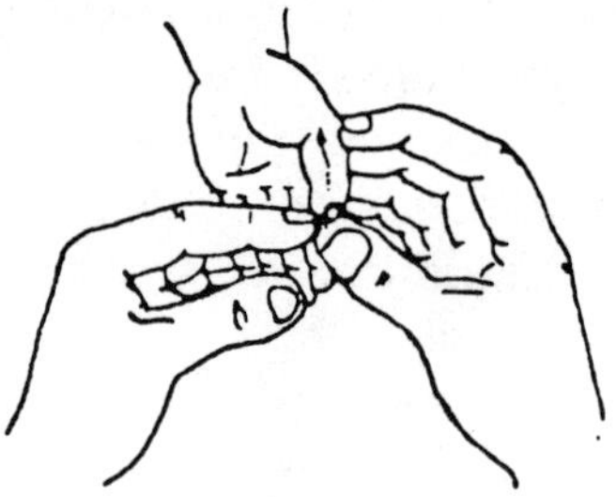

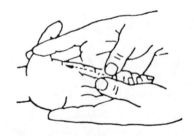

**Figure 14**

2. Rub the line on the lateral palmar side of the index finger, pushing in one direction only from the tip to the base of the index finger 100-300 times. (Fig. 15) This point is called *Da Chang Jing* (Large Intestine Channel) and this maneuver is referred to as supplementing the Large Intestine Channel. Stimulation of this point in this manner supplements the large intestine.

**Figure 15**

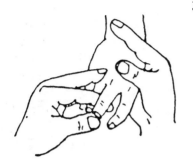

**Figure 16**

3. Knead the point on the center of the back of the hand 100-300 times. (Fig. 16)This point is called *Wai Lao Gong* (Outer Palace of Labor) and the movement is technically called kneading the Outer Palace of Labor. Stimulation of this point warms yang and disperses pathogenic cold.

4. Rub the line on the lateral edge of the anterior surface of the forearm, pushing in one direction only from the wrist to the elbow 100-300 times. (Fig. 17) This point is called *San Guan* (the Three Gates) and this maneuver is called straight pushing the Three Gates. Stimulation of this point warms yang and disperses pathogenic cold.

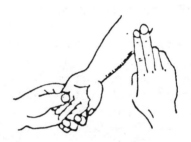

**Figure 17**

5. Round rub the abdomen around the navel counterclockwise from the practitioner's perspective. Do this with the hollow of the palm 100-500 times. (Fig. 18) This point is called *Fu* (the Abdomen) in Chinese, and this manipulation is called round rubbing the Abdomen. Stimulation of this point in this manner improves digestion and harmonizes the stomach and intestines.

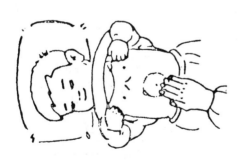

**Figure 18**

6. Rub the line on the center of the sacrum, pushing in one direction only from the tailbone to the small of the back 100-300 times. (Fig. 19) This point is called *Qi Jie Gu* (Seven Bound Bones, *i.e.*, the sacrum) and the maneuver is referred to by *tui na* practitioners as pushing the Sacrum. Stimulation of this point in this manner stops diarrhea.

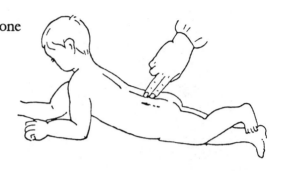

**Figure 19**

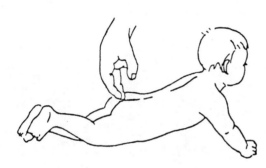

**Figure 20**

7. Knead the point under the tip of the tailbone with the tip of the middle finger 100-300 times. (Fig. 20) This point is called *Gui Wei* (Turtle Tail) and this manipulation is called kneading the Turtle's Tail. Stimulation of this point stops diarrhea.

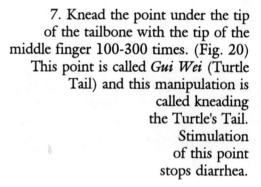

8. Knead the point below the knee on the lateral side of the lower leg between the tibia and fibula 50-100 times on both legs. (Fig. 21) This corresponds to the point *Zu San Li* (St 36) in acupuncture. This maneuver is, therefore, called kneading the Three *Li*. Stimulation of this point harmonizes the stomach and intestines and improves digestion.

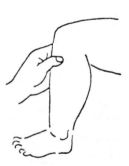

**Figure 21**

# Damp heat pattern (*shi re xing*)

**Disease causes:** This type of diarrhea most commonly occurs during hot or hot, damp weather in the late spring, summer, and early fall. It can also be caused eating spoiled or unclean food. In older children, it can be caused by overeating greasy foods, such as peanut butter, chips, hamburgers, pizza, french fries, etc.

**Main signs & symptoms:** Abdominal pain followed by loose, possibly explosive stools, yellowish brown or watery stools, possible mucus in the stools, offensively smelling stools, possible fever or body heat, thirst, dark, scanty urine, and a red anus with a burning feeling on defecation

**Treatment principles:** Clear heat, eliminate dampness, and stop diarrhea

**Treatment methods:**

1. Slightly stretch out the child's thumb and rub the line on the lateral palmar edge of the thumb, pushing in one direction only from the base to the tip 100-300 times. (Fig. 22) As mentioned above, this is point is called *Pi Jing* (Spleen Channel). This manipulation is called slightly draining the Spleen Channel. Stimulation of this point in this manner clears heat and eliminates dampness from the spleen, stomach, and intestines.

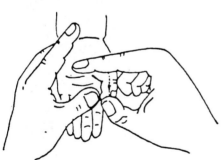

**Figure 22**

29

2. Rub the line on the lateral palmar surface of the index finger, pushing from the base to the tip 100-300 times. (Fig. 23) This is called slightly draining Large Intestine Channel. Stimulation of this point in this manner drains pathogens from the large intestine.

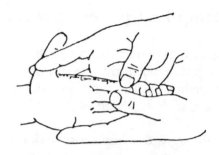

**Figure 23**

3. Rub the line on the medial (*i.e.*, ulnar), palmar edge of the little finger, pushing from the base to the tip 100-300 times. (Fig. 24) This point is called *Xiao Chang Jing* (Small Intestine Channel) and *tui na* practitioners refer to this maneuver as slightly draining the Small Intestine Channel. Stimulation of this point in this manner drains pathogens from the small intestine.

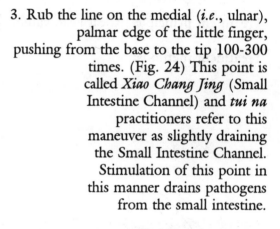

**Figure 24**

4. Rub the line on the midline of the anterior surface of the forearm, pushing from the wrist to the elbow, in one direction only 100-300 times. (Fig. 25) This point is called *Tian He Shui* (Heavenly Peace Water, *i.e.*, the Milky Way). The manipulation is, therefore, technically referred to as straight pushing the Milky Way. Stimulation of this point clears pathogenic heat.

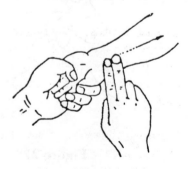

**Figure 25**

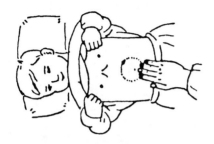

5. Round rub the abdomen around the navel clockwise with the hollow of the palm 100-500 times. (Fig. 26) This is called round rubbing the Abdomen. Round rubbing the Abdomen in this direction drains pathogens from the stomach and intestines.

**Figure 26**

6. Rub the line on the center of the sacrum, pushing from the small of the back to the tailbone 100-300 times. (Fig. 27) This is called pushing the Sacrum. Stimulation of this point in this manner drains pathogens from the intestines.

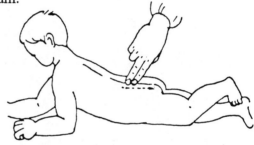

**Figure 27**

# Food damage pattern (*shang shi xing*)

**Disease causes:** This type of pediatric diarrhea is caused by overfeeding the baby or feeding the baby hard to digest foods. Because the baby's digestive tract is immature, it is important not to overfeed infants or to feed them hard to digest foods. It may also be caused by eating spoiled food or changing to an unfamiliar food or milk.

**Main signs & symptoms:** Copious stools with a rotten egg smell, abdominal pain relieved after emptying the bowels, abdominal distention or bloating, bad breath, and poor appetite

31

**Treatment principles:** Eliminate food stagnation and transform accumulations

**Treatment methods:**

1. Slightly stretch out the child's thumb and rub the line on the lateral palmar surface of the thumb, pushing from the tip to the base of the thumb 100-500 times. (Fig. 28) This is called supplementing the Spleen Channel. Stimulation of this point in this manner supplements the spleen and harmonizes the stomach and intestines.

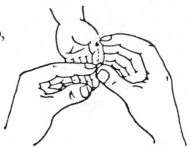

**Figure 28**

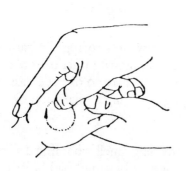

**Figure 29**

2. Rub the line on the lateral palmar surface of the index finger, pushing from the base to the tip 100-300 times. (Fig. 29) This is called slightly reducing the Large Intestine Channel. Stimulation of this point in this manner drains pathogens from the large intestine.

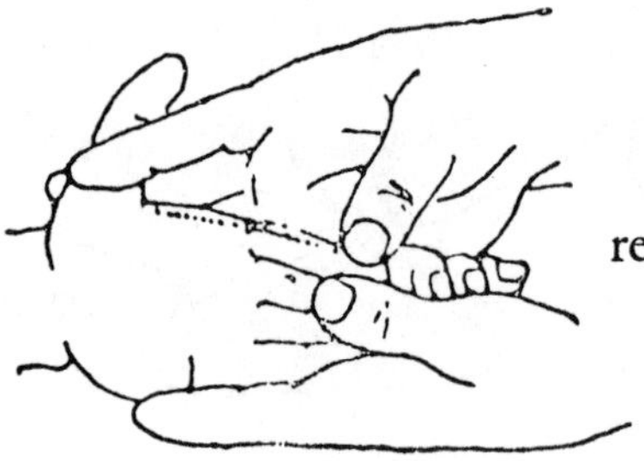

3. Rub the circle of the palm 100-300 times. The center of this circle is the center of the palm and its radius is 2/3 the length from the center of the palm to the transverse crease at the base of the middle finger. (Fig. 30) This point is called *Ba Gua* (the Eight Trigrams). This movement is called moving or transporting the Eight Trigrams. Stimulation of this point rectifies and frees the flow of qi and blood as well as harmonizes the functions of the five major organs.

**Figure 30**

4. Knead the large bulge at the base of the thumb 100-300 times. (Fig. 31) This is called the thenar eminence in Western anatomy and *Ban Men* (Shuttered Gate) in Chinese. Thus this manipulation is called kneading the Shuttered Gate. Stimulation of this point in this manner removes food stagnation and promotes digestion as well as drains replete heat in the spleen and stomach.

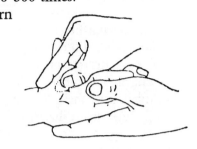

**Figure 31**

5. With both thumbs, obliquely push apart along the underside of the lower ribs from the upper belly to the sides of the abdomen 100-300 times. (Fig. 32) This manipulation is called pushing apart the Abdomen. Stimulation of this point in this manner strengthens the spleen and promotes digestion.

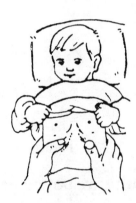

**Figure 32**

6. Round rub the abdomen around the navel clockwise with the hollow of the palm 100-500 times. (Fig. 33) This is called round rubbing the Abdomen. Stimulation of this point in this manner promotes digestion.

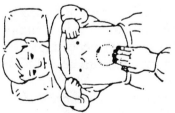

**Figure 33**

7. Rub the line on the center of the sacrum, pushing in one direction only from the tailbone upward to the small of the back 100-300 times. (Fig. 34) This is called pushing the Sacrum. Stimulation of this point in this manner stops diarrhea.

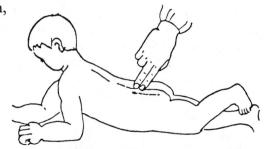

**Figure 34**

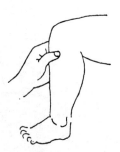

8. Knead the point located below the knee on the lateral side of the lower leg between the tibia and fibula 50-100 times on both legs. (Fig. 35) This is called kneading the Three *Li*. Stimulation of this point harmonizes the stomach and intestines and promotes digestion.

**Figure 35**

## Vacuity weakness pattern (*xu ruo xing*)

**Disease causes:** If diarrhea persists for a long time it can weaken the digestive system. The digestive system may also be weakened by chronic disease or may be constitutionally weak from birth.

**Main signs & symptoms:** Frequent, repeated bouts of diarrhea or protracted, unstoppable bouts of diarrhea, thin, light or white colored stools with lumps of undigested milk or containing undigested food, bowel movements immediately after eating, a sallow complexion, emaciation, poor appetite, and fatigue and listlessness

**Treatment principles:** Supplement the spleen, harmonize the stomach, and stop diarrhea

**Treatment methods:**
1. Slightly bend the child's thumb and rub the line on the lateral palmar surface of the thumb, pushing in one direction only from the tip to the base of the thumb 100-500 times. (Fig. 36) This is called supplementing the Spleen Channel. Stimulation of this point in this manner strengthens the spleen.

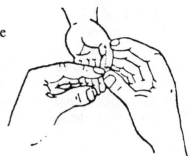

2. Rub the line on the lateral palmar surface of the index finger, pushing in one direction only from the tip to the base of the index finger 100-300 times. (Fig. 37) This is called supplementing the Large Intestine Channel. Stimulation of this point in this manner supplements the large intestine.

**Figure 37**

3. Rub the circle on the palm 100-300 times. This circle's center is the center of the palm and its radius is 2/3 the length from the center of the palm to the transverse crease at the base of the middle finger. (Fig. 38) This is called moving the Eight Trigrams. Stimulation of this point in this manner rectifies and frees the flow of the qi and blood as well as harmonizes the functions of the five major organs.

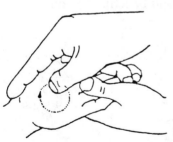

**Figure 38**

4. Round rub the abdomen around the navel counterclockwise with the hollow of the palm 100-500 times. (Fig. 39) This is called round rubbing the Abdomen. Stimulating this point in this manner supplements the center and strengthens the spleen.

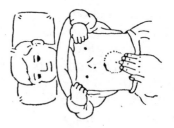

**Figure 39**

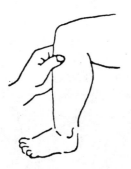

**Figure 40**

5. Knead the point below the knee on the lateral side of the lower leg between the tibia and fibula 50-100 times on both legs. (Fig. 40) This is called kneading Three *Li*. Stimulation of this point harmonizes the stomach and intestines and promotes digestion.

6. First apply some massage medium to the child's back. Massage lightly along the middle of the spine from above to below 3 times. Then put the hands on each side of the tailbone. Grasp and lift the skin with the thumbs and index and middle fingers of both hands, rolling the skin upward from the base of the tailbone to the base of the neck 3-5 times. (Fig. 41) This is called pinching and pulling the Spine. It strengthens the righteous qi of the entire body and benefits the constitution.

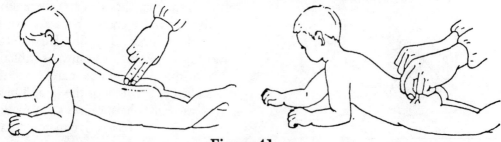

**Figure 41**

# Fright pattern (*jing xing*)

**Disease causes:** This type of diarrhea is caused by fright or emotional stress.

**Main signs & symptoms:** Small amounts of green, foamy stool, easy fright startling, difficulty sleeping, and morbid night-crying

**Treatment principles:** Supplement the spleen, clear the heart, and quiet the spirit

**Treatment methods:**

1. Slightly bend the child's thumb and rub the line on the lateral palmar surface of the thumb, pushing in one direction only from the tip to the base of the thumb 100-500 times. (Fig. 42) This is called supplementing the Spleen Channel. Stimulating this point in this manner strengthens the spleen and supplements the middle.

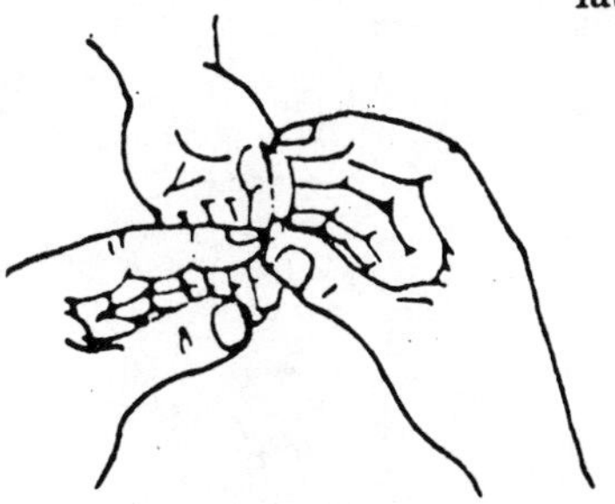

**Figure 42**

2. Rub the line on the lateral palmar surface of the index finger, pushing in one direction only from the tip to the base of the index finger 100-300 times. (Fig. 43) This is called supplementing the Large Intestine Channel. Stimulation of this point in this manner supplements the large intestine.

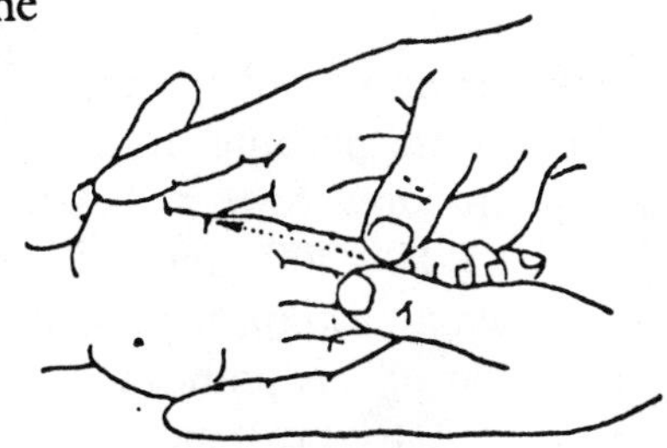

**Figure 43**

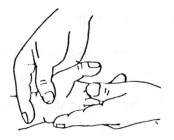

**Figure 44**

3. Nip and knead the point at the midpoint of the base of the palm where the major and minor bulges of the palm meet below the crease of the wrist. Nip 3-5 times and knead 50-100 times. (Fig. 44) This point is called *Xiao Tian Xin* (Small Heavenly Heart). This maneuver is called nipping and kneading the Small Heavenly Heart. Stimulation of this point quiets the spirit and stops fright.

4. Round rub the abdomen around the navel from right to left or counterclockwise from the therapist's perspective. Do this with the hollow of the palm 100-500 times. (Fig. 45) This is called round rubbing the Abdomen. Stimulation of this point in this manner strengthens the digestion and harmonizes the stomach and intestines.

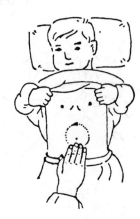

**Figure 45**

5. Rub the line on the center of the sacrum, pushing from the tailbone upward to the small of the back 100-300 times. (Fig. 46) This is called pushing the Sacrum. Stimulation of this point in this manner stops diarrhea.

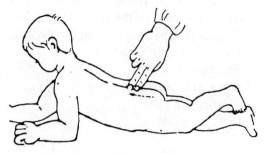

**Figure 46**

6. Apply some massage medium to the child's back. Then lightly massage along the middle of the spine from above to below 3-5 times. Next put the hands on each side of the tailbone and grasp and lift the skin with the thumbs and the index and middle fingers of both hands, rolling the skin upward from the tailbone to the base of the neck 3-5 times. (Fig. 47) This is called pinching and pulling the Spine. Stimulation of this point strengthens the constitution and supports the righteous qi.

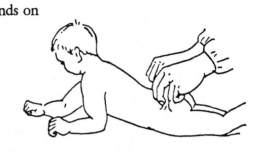

**Figure 47**

## Points for Special Attention

**1.** Children suffering from diarrhea should be given easily digestible food and should not be overfed. for more information on the feeding of infants and children according to TCM theory, the reader should see Bob Flaws' *Arisal of the Clear: A Simple Guide to Healthy Eating According to Traditional Chinese Medicine* and his *Food, Phlegm, and Pediatric Disease,* both available from Blue Poppy Press.

**2.** Most children with diarrhea do not need to take any medication unless they have epidemic or infectious diarrhea. In that case, if the diarrhea is serious and accompanied by fever and if a stool test reveals the presence of many white blood cells, the child can take medicine for a few days combined with the above appropriate massage therapy.

**3.** If a child with diarrhea does not recover after prolonged administration of medicine, the medication should be stopped and the child should be treated by massage only. This is because the medicine, such as certain antibiotics, may actually be causing or aggravating the diarrhea.

**4.** One should pay close attention to what is called physiological diarrhea. This kind of diarrhea occurs soon after birth. In this case, there are bowel movements 3-7 times per day which are yellowish green in color. Otherwise the child has good spirits and appetite and their growth is normal. Most children with this kind of diarrhea are breastfed. In such cases, the mother's milk is clearer than usual. This condition does not respond to either medicine or massage. The only method capable of treating it is to add supplementary food earlier than otherwise recommended. The baby will recover after suitable adjustments have been made to their diet.

**5.** The above massage protocols are typically performed only once per day. however, if the child's condition is serious, it may be performed twice per day.

# CHAPTER 2

# Abdominal Pain

Abdominal pain is a common pediatric symptom accompanying a variety of illnesses. The treatments suggested below are suitable for most types of childhood abdominal pain. However, it should not be used for the treatment of abdominal pain caused by acute abdominal diseases, such as appendicitis. In particular, the protocols given below are very effective for the treatment of pediatric colic. This consists of abdominal pain in infants which occurs daily in the late afternoon and lasts into the evening or throughout the night. Colic may begin either a few days or a few weeks after birth and can last for three months if left untreated.

In order to know if their infant or very young child has abdominal pain, parents must observe their child carefully. Since infants and young children cannot verbalize their feelings adequately, they express their discomfort in other ways. A contorted, pained facial expression, pulling the legs back toward the belly, crying with the back arched backwards, and continuing to cry even after their diaper has been changed all suggest the presence of abdominal pain.

## Patterns & Their Treatment

### Cold pattern (*han xing*)

**Disease causes:** This type of abdominal pain is caused by eating cold foods and cold drinks and by cold weather. It can easily be cured by pediatric *tui na*.

**Main signs & symptoms:** Sudden abdominal pain, crying in pain, abdominal pain which is more severe after exposure to cold or after eating cold, raw foods or drinking cold drinks, abdominal pain which is comforted by warming the belly, a soft, atonic abdomen, a darkish but nonetheless pale complexion, possible diarrhea or watery stool, and light colored, paler than normal urination

**Treatment principles:** Warm yang, disperse cold, and relieve pain

**Treatment methods:**

1. Slightly bend the child's thumb and rub the line on the lateral palmar surface of the thumb, pushing in one direction only from the tip to the base of the thumb 100-500 times. (Fig. 48) This is called supplementing the Spleen Channel. Stimulation of this point in this manner strengthens the spleen and supplements the center (*i.e.*, digestion).

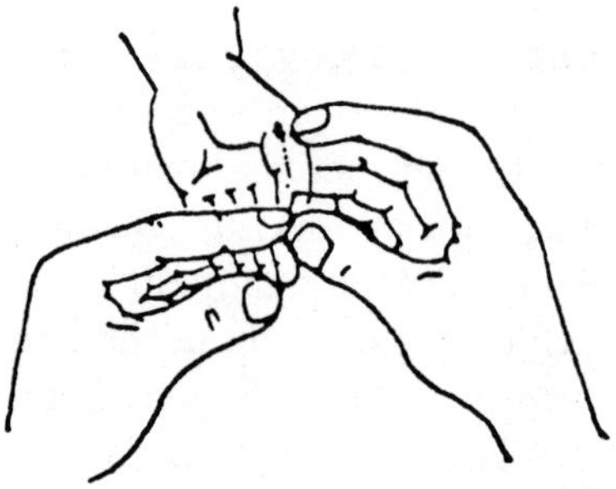

**Figure 48**

2. Knead the point on the center of the back of the hand 100-300 times. (Fig. 49) This is called kneading the Outer Palace of Labor. Stimulation of this point warms yang and disperses pathogenic cold. In particular, it warms the lower burner.

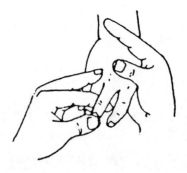

**Figure 49**

3. Knead the point at the middle of the crease of the wrist on the back or posterior side of the hand 100-300 times. (Fig. 50) This point is called *Yi Wo Feng* ([Number] One Nest of Wind). This maneuver is thus called kneading the Number One Nest of Wind by *tui na* practitioners. Stimulation of this point warms the middle burner, moves the qi, and relieves abdominal pain.

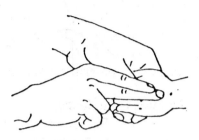

**Figure 50**

4. Rub the line on the lateral edge of the anterior surface of the forearm, pushing in one direction only from the wrist to the elbow 100-300 times. (Fig. 51) This point is called *San Guan* (Three Gates or Barriers), and this manipulation is called straight pushing the Three Gates. Stimulating this point supplements the qi and fortifies yang as well as disperses pathogenic cold.

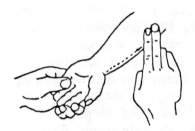

**Figure 51**

5. Round rub the abdomen around the navel from right to left or counterclockwise from the therapist's perspective. Do this with the hollow of the palm 100-500 times. (Fig. 52) This is called round rubbing the Abdomen. Stimulating this point in this manner supplements the center (*i.e.*, strengthens digestion) and harmonizes the stomach and intestines.

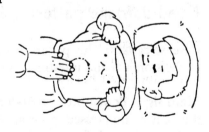

**Figure 52**

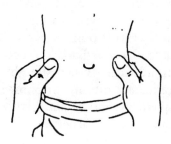

6. Knead the point below the knee on the lateral side of the lower leg between the tibia and fibula 50-100 times on both legs. (Fig. 53) This is called kneading Three *Li*. Stimulation of this point supplements the center and harmonizes the stomach and intestines.

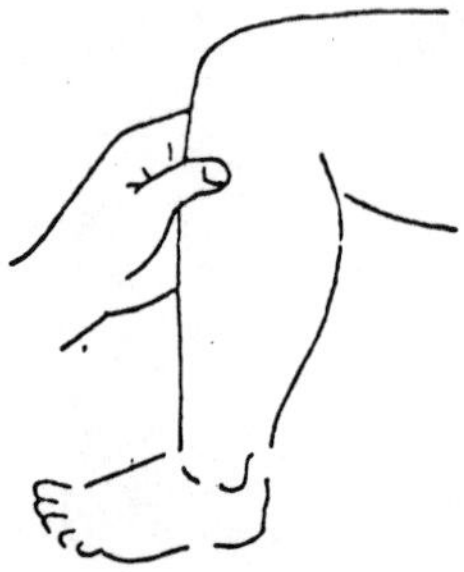

**Figure 53**

7. Grasp and lift the abdominal muscles at both sides of the abdomen at the level of the navel. Grasp and lift with the thumbs and index and middle fingers of both hands 3-5 times. (Fig. 54) This point is called *Du Jiao* (Triple Angles, *i.e.*, the angles of the intestines). This maneuver is called grasping the Angles of the Intestines. Stimulation of this point stops abdominal pain.

**Figure 54**

## Food damage pattern (*shang shi xing*)

**Disease causes:** This pattern is due to overfeeding of infants. Thus food stagnates in the stomach and intestines causing distention and pain.

**Main signs & symptoms:** Abdominal pain with distention, unwillingness to allow the belly to be pressed, poor appetite, burping with a foul smell or vomiting food with a foul smell, frequent flatulence, diarrhea with a rotten egg smell or constipation, and less pain after bowel movements

**Treatment principles:** Eliminate food stagnation, transform accumulations, and relieve pain

**Treatment methods:**

1. Slightly bend the child's thumb and rub the line on the lateral palmar edge of the thumb, pushing in one direction only from the tip to the base of the thumb 100-500 times. (Fig. 55) This is called supplementing the Spleen Channel. Stimulation of this point in this manner strengthens the spleen and supplements the center, thus promoting digestion.

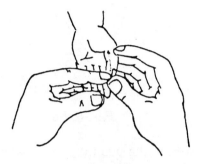

**Figure 55**

2. Rub the line on the lateral palmar edge of the index finger, pushing in one direction only from the base of the finger to the tip 100-300 times. (Fig. 56) This is called slightly draining the Large Intestine Channel. Stimulation of this point in this manner drains the large intestine and removes accumulated (undigested) food.

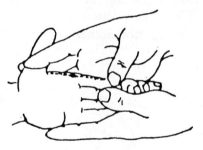

**Figure 56**

3. Knead the thenar eminence or major bulge at the base of the thumb 100-300 times. (Fig. 57) This is called kneading the Shuttered Gate. Stimulation of this point removes accumulated food in the stomach, promotes digestion, and drains replete heat in the spleen and stomach.

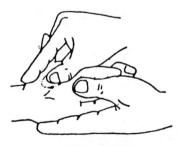

**Figure 57**

**45**

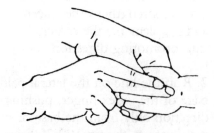

4. Rub the circle on the palm 100-300 times. This circle's center is the center of the palm and its radius is 2/3 the length from the center of the palm to the transverse crease at the base of the middle finger. (Fig. 58) This is called moving or transporting the Eight Trigrams. Stimulation of this point in this manner moves and quickens the qi and blood as well as harmonizes the functions of the five major organs.

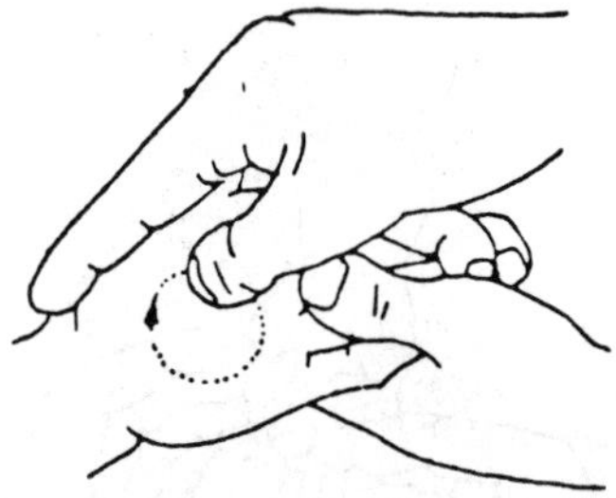

**Figure 58**

5. Knead the point on the back of the wrist in the middle of the transverse crease 100-300 times. (Fig. 59) This manipulation is called kneading the Number One Nest of Wind. Stimulation of this point stops abdominal pain.

**Figure 59**

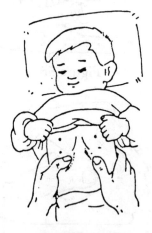

6. With both thumbs, obliquely push apart in one direction only along the underside of the ribs from the upper belly to the sides of the abdomen 100-300 times. (Fig. 60) This manipulation is called pushing apart the Abdomen. Stimulation of this point strengthens the spleen and stomach and promotes digestion.

**Figure 60**

7. Knead the point above the navel with the hollow of the palm of the hand clockwise 100-300 times. (Fig. 61) This point is called *Zhong Wan* (Central Venter). *Zhong Wan* is the name of acupuncture point CV 12. This maneuver is referred to as kneading the Central Venter by *tui na* practitioners. Stimulation of this point in this manner strengthens the spleen and stomach and promotes digestion.

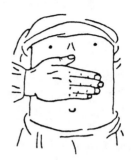

**Figure 61**

8. Knead the point below the knee on the lateral side of the lower leg between the tibia and fibula. Do this 50-100 times on both sides. (Fig. 62) This is called kneading Three *Li*. Stimulation of this point harmonizes the stomach and intestines and promotes digestion.

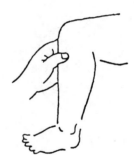

**Figure 62**

9. Grasp and lift the abdominal muscles at both sides of the abdomen at the level of the navel. Grasp and lift with the thumbs and index and middle fingers of both hands 3-5 times. (Fig. 63) This is called grasping the Angles of the Intestines. Stimulation of this point relieves abdominal pain.

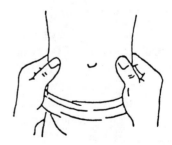

**Figure 63**

# Vacuity weakness pattern (*xu ruo xing*)

**Disease causes:** This may be due to constitutional weakness in the infant.

**Main signs & symptoms:** Dull abdominal pain which feels better with both warmth and pressure, a soft, atonic belly, a sallow, sickly complexion, emaciation, poor appetite, and a tendency to diarrhea

**Treatment principles:** Supplement the spleen, harmonize the stomach, and relieve pain

**Treatment methods:**

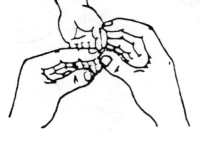

1. Slightly bend the child's thumb and rub the line on the lateral palmar edge of the thumb, pushing in one direction only from the tip to the base of the thumb 100-500 times. (Fig. 64) This is called supplementing the Spleen Channel. Stimulation of this point in this manner strengthens the spleen and supplements the center, thus promoting digestion.

**Figure 64**

2. Rub the line on the medial side of the palmar surface of the little finger and medial edge of the palm, pushing from the base of the palm to the tip of the small finger 100-500 times. (Fig. 65) This is called fortifying the Kidney Channel. Stimulation of this point in this manner supplements the kidneys and strengthens the body.

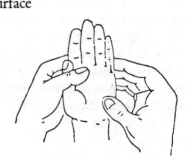

**Figure 65**

3. Knead the point in the center of the back of the hand 100-300 times. (Fig. 66) This is called kneading the Outer Palace of Labor. Stimulation of this point warms yang and disperses pathogenic cold. In particular, it warms the lower burner.

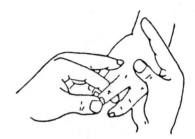

**Figure 66**

4. Knead the point at the middle of the crease of the wrist on the back of the hand 100-300 times. (Fig. 67) This is called kneading the Number One Nest of Wind. Stimulation of this point warms the middle burner, moves the qi, and relieves abdominal pain.

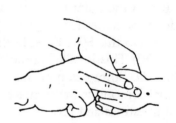

**Figure 67**

5. Rub the line on the lateral side of the anterior of the forearm, pushing from the wrist to the elbow 100-300 times. (Fig. 68) This is called straight pushing the Three Gates. Stimulation of this point warms yang and disperses pathogenic cold.

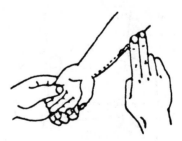

**Figure 68**

**49**

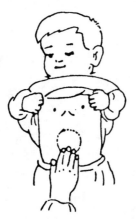

**Figure 69**

6. Round rub the abdomen around the navel from right to left or counterclockwise from the practitioner's perspective. Do this with the hollow of the palm 100-500 times. (Fig. 69) This is called round rubbing the Abdomen. Stimulation of this point in this manner supplements the center and strengthens the digestion.

7. Knead the point below the knee on the lateral side of the lower leg between the tibia and fibula. Do this 50-100 on both legs. (Fig. 70) This is called kneading Three *Li*. Stimulation of this point harmonizes the stomach and intestines and promotes digestion.

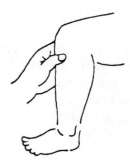

**Figure 70**

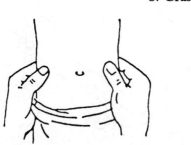

**Figure 71**

8. Grasp and lift the abdominal muscles at both sides of the abdomen at the level of the navel. Grasp and lift with the thumbs and index and middle fingers of both hands 3-5 times. (Fig. 71) This is called grasping the Angles of the Intestines. Stimulation of this point relieves abdominal pain.

9. First apply some massage medium to the child's back and massage lightly along the middle of the spine from above to below 3 times. Then place the hands on each side of the tailbone. Grasp and lift the skin with the thumbs and index and middle fingers of both hands, rolling the skin upward from the tailbone to the base of the neck 3-5 times. (Fig. 72) This is called pinching and pulling the Spine. Stimulation of this point in this way strengthens the constitution and supports the righteous qi of the body.

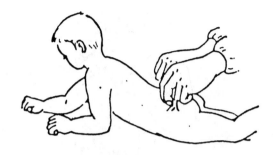

**Figure 72**

# Worms (*chong*)

**Disease causes:** Worms in TCM are believed to be caused by damp heat in the stomach and intestines, in turn developing due to weak spleen and stomach function. Obviously, they also have to do with food sanitation.

**Main signs & symptoms:** Abrupt, intermittent abdominal pain, especially around the navel, reduction of pain by pressing or kneading the belly, wriggling lumps can be seen in the abdomen, massaged, and then disappear, possible appearance of worms in the stools, loss of weight or emaciation, poor appetite, grinding of teeth in sleep at night, eating of non-food substances, such as dirt, ashes, etc., and occasional vomiting

**Treatment principles:** Transform and expel worms, relieve pain

**Treatment methods:**

1. Slightly bend the child's thumb and rub the line on the lateral palmar edge of the

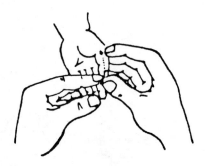

**Figure 73**

thumb, pushing in one direction only from the tip to the base of the thumb 100-500 times. (Fig. 73) This is called supplementing the Spleen Channel. Stimulation of this point in this manner strengthens the spleen and supplements the center, thus strengthening digestion.

2. Knead the point on the center of the back of the hand 100-300 times. (Fig. 74) This is called kneading the Outer Palace of Labor. Stimulating this point warms the yang and disperses cold. In particular, it warms the lower burner.

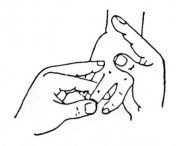

**Figure 74**

3. Knead the point at the middle of the transverse crease on the back of the wrist 100-300 times. (Fig. 75) This is called kneading the Number One Nest of Wind. Stimulating warms the center, moves the qi, and relieves abdominal pain.

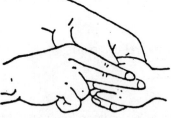

**Figure 75**

4. Rub the line on the lateral anterior surface of the forearm from the wrist to the elbow 100-300 times. (Fig. 76) This is called straight pushing the Three Gates. Stimulating this point warms yang and disperses pathogenic cold.

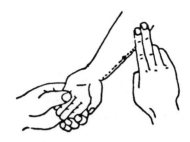

**Figure 76**

5. Knead the navel clockwise with the hollow of the palm 100-300 times. (Fig. 77) The navel is called *Qi*. Therefore, this manipulation is called kneading the Navel. Stimulation of this point warms yang and supplements vacuity, particularly spleen vacuity weakness.

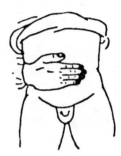

**Figure 77**

## Points for Special Attention

1. If the child has serious abdominal pain and abnormal complexion, the parents should take care to discriminate if the child's condition is one of several acute abdominal diseases, such as appendicitis, intestinal obstruction, and intussusception. Acute abdominal diseases have two main characteristics:

   **A.** The abdominal pain is continuous and exists as long as the pathological condition does. Some diseases are accompanied by abdominal angina. Abdominal angina means the occlusion or obstruction of the arteries in the abdomen resulting cramplike pain, especially after eating, possible constipation, occasional

**53**

melena or dark blood in the stools, progressive weight loss, and malabsorption syndrome.

**B.** The place of pain is fixed. The quality of the pain is pressing. There is tightness of the abdominal muscles, possible wriggling lumps, or the intestines may wiggle in waves. The characteristics of appendicitis are pressing pain on the right, lower abdomen accompanied by fever. The characteristics of intestinal obstruction are frequent, copious vomiting, loud, sonorous rumbling of the intestines, and intestinal wriggling. The characteristics of intussusception are morbid crying, the presence of a palpable lump, and jam-like blood in the stool.

If any of the above symptoms are found, the child should be hospitalized immediately.

**2.** Children with abdominal pain due to parasites should be treated with medication to kill the worms after the abdominal pain has been relieved by *tui na.*

**3.** In general, avoid feeding children raw, cold, frozen, refrigerated, or unclean foods and drinks.

**4.** Typically massage for the treatment of abdominal pain should be performed once per day. However, if the condition is severe, it may be done twice per day. Most commonly, children with abdominal pain treated by pediatric *tui na* recover after 1-3 days of treatment.

CHAPTER 3

# Vomiting

V omiting is a symptom accompanying many childhood illnesses. Because children's digestive function is immature and, therefore, inherently weak as compared to an adult's, vomiting is most often caused by inappropriate feeding or foods or adverse climatic factors. Western medical diagnoses accounting for pediatric vomiting most often are gastritis and indigestion. Treatment with Chinese infant massage is most definitely effective for these kinds of vomiting.

If, after being fed milk, the baby has milk dribbling from the corner of his or her mouth, this is called milk overflow. The cardia of the stomach in the baby is more flaccid than in the adult. If inappropriately fed or overfed with milk or much air is gulped down while eating, the nursing infant may often have milk overflow. This is not a cause for alarm, nor is it a disease. It can be stopped by lightly patting the baby's back.

## Patterns & Their Treatment

### Cold pattern (*han xing*)

**Disease causes:** These are the same as discussed under this heading in the previous two diseases.

**Main signs & symptoms:** Vomiting immediately after eating, however the vomitus is not particularly fetid smelling, a pale complexion, cold extremities, accompanying abdominal pain is reduced by warmth applied to the belly, and possible watery diarrhea

**Treatment principles:** Warm yang, disperse cold, descend counterflow, and stop vomiting

**Treatment methods:**

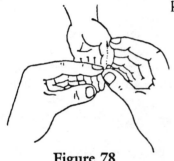

**Figure 78**

1. Slightly bend the child's thumb and rub the line on the lateral palmar edge of the thumb, pushing in one direction only from the tip to the base of the thumb 100-500 times. (Fig. 78) This is called supplementing the Spleen Channel. Stimulating this point in this manner strengthens the spleen and supplements center, thus strengthening digestion.

2. Rub the line on the thenar eminence or major bulge at the base of the thumb, pushing from the crease of the wrist to the base of the thumb 100-300 times. (Fig. 79) This is called pushing *Heng Wen* (Horizontal Crease) to *Ban Men* (Shuttered Gate). Stimulation of this point relieves stuffiness in the chest and abdomen and relieves vomiting.

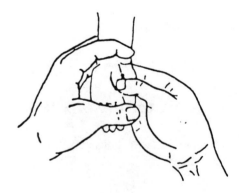

**Figure 79**

3. Knead the point in the center of the back of the hand 100-300 times. (Fig. 80) This is called kneading Outer Palace of Labor. Stimulation of this point warms yang and disperses cold and, in particular, warms the lower burner.

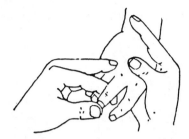

**Figure 80**

4. Rub the line on the lateral anterior surface of the forearm, pushing in one direction only from the wrist to the elbow and in that direction only 100-300 times. (Fig. 81) This is called straight pushing the Three Gates. Stimulation of this point warms yang and disperses cold.

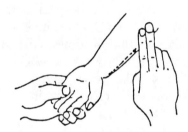

**Figure 81**

5. Knead the point above the navel at the midpoint of the upper abdomen clockwise with the hollow of the palm 100-300 times. (Fig. 82) This is called kneading the Central Venter. Stimulation of this point relieves vomiting and strengthens the spleen and stomach.

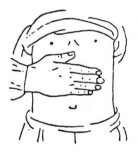

**Figure 82**

57

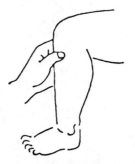

**Figure 83**

6. Knead the point below the knee on the lateral edge of the lower leg between the tibia and the fibula. (Fig. 83) This is called kneading Three *Li*. Stimulation of this point harmonizes the stomach and intestines and promotes digestion.

7. Rub the back of the neck, pushing in one direction only from the hairline to the bulging bone (C7) at the base of the neck 100-500 times. (Fig. 84) This point is called *Tian Zhu Gu* (Heavenly Pillar Bones) and this maneuver is called pushing the Heavenly Pillar Bones. Stimulation of this point promotes the downward descent of qi.

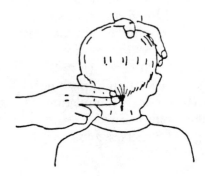

**Figure 84**

## Heat pattern (*re xing*)

**Disease causes:** The causes of this condition are similar to those discussed under damp heat pattern diarrhea.

**Main signs & symptoms:** Vomiting immediately after eating, putrid smelling vomitus, possible excessive body heat or fever, thirst, putrid smelling stools, and darker than normal urine

**Treatment principles:** Clear heat from the stomach, descend counterflow, and stop vomiting

**Treatment methods:**

1. Rub the line on the lateral palmar edge of
the thumb, pushing in one direction
only from the base to the tip of
thumb 100-300 times. (Fig. 85)
This is called slightly
draining the Spleen
Channel. Stimulation of
this point in this manner
drains repletion from
the spleen and stomach.

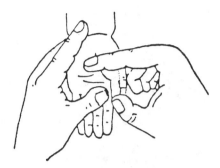

**Figure 85**

2. Rub the line on the lateral palmar edge of
the index finger, pushing in one direction only
from the base to the tip of the index finger 100-300
times. (Fig. 86) This is called
slightly draining the Large Intestine
Channel. Stimulation of this point
clears heat from the large
intestine and drains repletion.

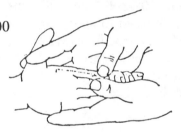

**Figure 86**

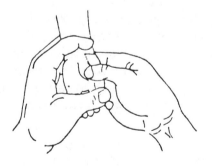

**Figure 87**

3. Rub the line on the thenar eminence or major
bulge at the base of the thumb, pushing
from the wrist to the base of the
thumb 100-300 times. (Fig. 87) This is
called pushing from the Horizontal Crease
to the Shuttered Gate. Stimulation of this
point relieves stuffiness in the chest and
abdomen and relieves vomiting.

59

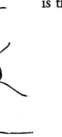

**Figure 88**

4. Rub the circle on the palm 100-300 times. This circle's center is the center of the palm and its radius is 2/3 the length from the center to the transverse crease at the base of the middle finger. (Fig. 88) This is called moving or transporting the Eight Trigrams. Stimulation of this point in this manner moves and quickens the qi and blood and harmonizes the functions of the five major organs.

5. Rub the line on the middle of the anterior or palmar surface of the forearm, pushing from the wrist to the elbow 100-300 times. (Fig. 89) This is called straight pushing the Milky Way. Stimulation of this point clears heat and drains fire.

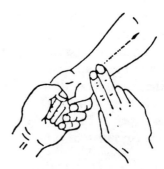

**Figure 89**

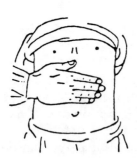

**Figure 90**

6. Knead the point above the navel in the center of the upper abdomen with the hollow of the palm 100-300 times. (Fig. 90) This is called kneading the Central Venter. Stimulation of this point relieves vomiting and strengthens the spleen and stomach.

7. Rub the line on the sacrum, pushing downward from the small of the back to the tailbone 100-300 times. (Fig. 91) This is called straight pushing the Sacrum. Stimulating this point in this manner disinhibits the bowels and promotes bowel movements, thus draining heat from the bowels.

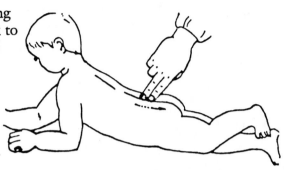

**Figure 91**

8. Rub the line on the back of the neck, pushing in one direction only from the hairline downward to the bulging bone (C7) at the base of the neck 100-500 times. (Fig. 92) This is called pushing the Heavenly Pillar Bones. Stimulation of this point promotes the downward descent of qi and relieves vomiting.

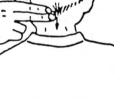

**Figure 92**

## Food damage pattern (*shang shi xing*)

**Disease causes:** Overfeeding or feeding difficult to digest food too early

**Main signs & symptoms:** Repeated, copious vomiting, sour, bad smelling vomitus including milky curds and undigested food, bad breath, poor appetite, abdominal distention and pain, diarrhea or constipation, and stool smelling like rotten eggs

**Treatment principles:** Eliminate food stagnation, transform accumulations, descend counterflow, and stop vomiting

**Treatment methods:**

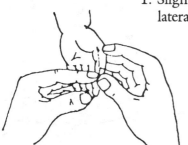

**Figure 93**

1. Slightly bend the child's thumb and the rub the line on the lateral palmar edge of the thumb, pushing in one direction only from the tip to the base of thumb 100-500 times. (Fig. 93) This is called supplementing the Spleen Channel. Stimulation of this point in this way strengthens the spleen and supplements the center, thus strengthening digestion.

2. Knead the thenar eminence or large bulge at the base of the thumb 100-300 times. (Fig. 94) This is called kneading the Shuttered Gate. Stimulation of this point removes accumulated food and promotes digestion at the same time as it clears replete heat from the spleen and stomach.

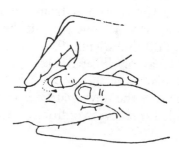

**Figure 94**

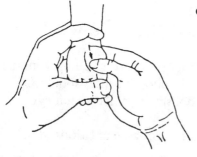

**Figure 95**

3. Rub the line on the thenar eminence or major bulge at the base of the thumb, pushing from the crease of the wrist to the base of the thumb 100-300 times. (Fig. 95) This is called pushing from the Horizontal Crease to the Shuttered Gate. Stimulation of this point relieves stuffiness in the chest and abdomen and relieves vomiting.

4. Rub the circle on the palm 100-300 times.
This circle's center is the center of
the palm and its radius is 2/3 the
length from the center of the palm
to the transverse crease at the
base of the middle finger. (Fig. 96)
This is called moving or transporting
the Eight Trigrams. Stimulating this
point in this manner moves and
quickens the qi and blood and
harmonizes the functions of the five major organs.

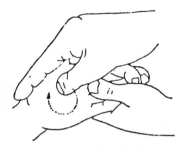

**Figure 96**

5. Knead the point above the navel
in the center of the upper
abdomen with the hollow of the palm
clockwise 100-300 times. (Fig. 97)
This is called kneading the Central
Venter. Stimulation of this point
in this manner promotes digestion
and relieves vomiting.

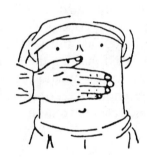

**Figure 97**

6. With both thumbs, obliquely push apart
along under the ribs from the upper
belly to the side of the abdomen 100-300
times. (Fig. 98) This is called
pushing apart the Abdomen.
Stimulation of this point
strengthens the spleen and
stomach and promotes digestion.

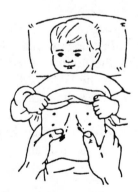

**Figure 98**

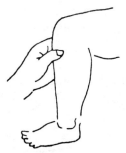

**Figure 99**

7. Knead the point below the knee on the lateral side of the lower leg between the tibia and fibula 50-100 times. (Fig. 99) This is called kneading Three *Li*. Stimulation of this point harmonizes the stomach and intestines and promotes digestion.

8. Rub the line on the back of the neck, pushing in one direction only downward from the hairline to the bulging bone (C7) at the base of the neck 100-500 times. (Fig. 100) This is called pushing the Heavenly Pillar Bones. Stimulation of this point promotes the downward descent of qi and relieves vomiting.

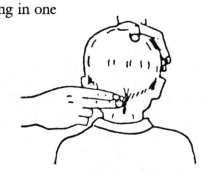

**Figure 100**

## Points for Special Attention

**1.** Babies with vomiting should be fed liquid or semi-liquid food that is easily digested. Feedings should be frequent but small in amount. Babies with serious vomiting should not be fed but should only be given dilute sugar water or saline solution. In the West pediatric electrolyte replacement liquids are available at drugstores over the counter.

**2.** Babies with vomiting should be made to lie on their right sides so as to prevent aspiration of vomitus and choking.

**3.** In case of serious vomiting with high fever and convulsion or with serious, drum-like abdominal distention and inability to pass gas, the baby should be taken to the hospital immediately,

**4.** As in the above pediatric diseases, for mild cases of vomiting, massage once per day. In serious cases, one can perform the above protocols twice per day.

CHAPTER

4

# Lack of Appetite

I n the case of lack of appetite, the child becomes tired of eating after eating only a little or refuses to eat at all. In China, this has become a common problem due to parents (who are more affluent and are only allowed to have one child) overfeeding their young charges. All parents want their children to be strong and healthy. Thus they put undue emphasis on highly nutritious, yet hard to digest food, such as meat, and feed their children rich food blindly, not realizing that children's digestion is much weaker than adults'. If the child overeats raw or chilled, frozen, cold foods or drinks, or greasy food, overeats in general or eats irregularly, the digestive function of the child will be dampened, causing loss of appetite.

The pediatric *tui na* treatment of lack of appetite is highly effective. Typically, children recover their normal appetite in one week.

**Disease causes:** Discussed above

**Main signs & symptoms:** Poor appetite, no desire to eat, or refusal to be fed, abdominal fullness and distention, indigestion, irregular bowel movements with foul odor, loss of weight, a dull, lusterless complexion, listlessness, possible slight fever, and restless sleep

**Treatment principles:** Supplement the spleen and harmonize the stomach, eliminate food stagnation and transform accumulations

**Treatment methods:**

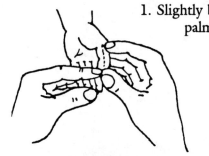

**Figure 101**

1. Slightly bend the child's thumb and rub the line on the lateral palmar edge of the thumb, pushing in one direction only from the tip to the base of the thumb 100-500 times. (Fig. 101) This is called supplementing the Spleen Channel. Stimulating this point in this manner strengthens the spleen and supplements the center, thus strengthening digestion.

2. Knead the thenar eminence or major bulge at the base of the thumb 100-300 times. (Fig. 102) This is called kneading the Shuttered Gate. Stimulation of this point dispels accumulated food and promotes digestion.

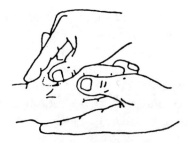

**Figure 102**

3. Rub the circle on the palm of the hand 100-300 times. This circle's center is the center of the palm and its radius is 2/3 the length of the center to the transverse crease at the base of the middle finger. (Fig. 103) This is called moving or transporting the Eight Trigrams. Stimulating this point in this manner moves and quickens the qi and blood and harmonizes the functions of the five major organs.

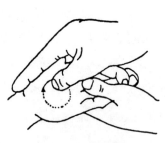

**Figure 103**

4. Nip and knead the points at the middle of the transverse creases on the palmar surfaces of the middle knuckles of the index, middle, ring, and little fingers. Nip 3-5 times each. Knead 30-50 times apiece. (Fig. 104) These points are called the *Si Heng Wen* (Four Horizontal Lines). Therefore, this maneuver is called nipping the Four Horizontal Lines. Stimulation of this point dispels stagnation and removes accumulated food.

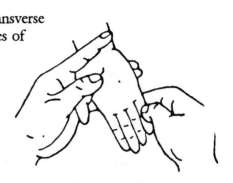

**Figure 104**

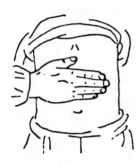

**Figure 105**

5. Knead the point above the navel in the center of the upper abdomen with the hollow of the palm clockwise 100-300 times. (Fig. 105) This is called kneading the Central Venter. Stimulating this point in this manner promotes digestion.

6. With both thumbs, obliquely push apart along the underside of the ribs from the upper abdomen to the sides of the abdomen 100-300 times. (Fig. 106) This is called pushing apart the Abdomen. Stimulation of this point strengthens the spleen and stomach and promotes digestion.

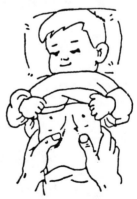

**Figure 106**

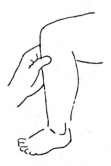

7. Knead the point below the knee on the lateral side of the lower leg between the tibia and fibula 50-100 times on both legs. (Fig. 107) This is called kneading Three *Li*. Stimulation of this point harmonizes the stomach and intestines and promotes digestion.

**Figure 107**

8. First apply some massage medium to the child's back. Then massage lightly along the middle of the spine from above to below 3 times. Putting the hands on each side of the sacrum, grasp and lift the skin with the thumbs and index and middle fingers, rolling the skin upward from the tailbone to the base of the neck 3-5 times. (Fig. 108) This is called pinching and pulling the Spine. Stimulating this point in this manner strengthens the constitution, supports the righteous qi, and improves the appetite.

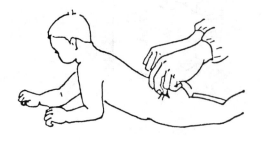

**Figure 108**

## Points for Special Attention

**1.** The child should be fed definite quantities of food at regular intervals. Thus the child will be neither too full nor too empty. One should not feed young children raw, cold, frozen, or chilled foods and drinks nor greasy, fatty, hard to digest foods.

**2.** Add additional food gradually as the child grows. Overfeeding sugar and sweets should be strictly avoided. Also, large quantities of a single food should not be given. All food should be freshly purchased or harvested, clean (*i.e.*, unsoiled or tainted), and freshly cooked.

**3.** Do not force a child to eat if he or she is unwilling as this may induce a psychological aversion to eating. Moreover, do not allow the child to form bad eating habits, such as reading or playing when eating.

**4.** The above massage protocol should be performed once per day with 6 treatments comprising one course of therapy. Typically, the child will be cured after a single such course. If the child is not completely cured in one course, another course should be continued after a 1-2 day rest.

# Constipation

Constipation refers to the child's inability to pass stool easily or comfortably. Constipation is a common pediatric complaint. The causes of constipation include:

## 1. Improper feeding

Since bowel movements are closely related to the diet, constipation may occur when:

**A.** The child eats too much high protein foods, such as eggs and milk;

**B.** The child eats highly refined foods with insufficient fiber, such as white flour products;

**C.** The child eats cold desserts, such as ice cream and frozen yogurt, or too many sugars and sweets.

## 2. Functional disorders of the intestinal tract

**A.** Irregular habits. Failure to empty the bowels regularly may cause the intestinal and abdominal muscles to lose their strength, thus causing constipation.

**B.** Chronic disease can cause functional disorder of the intestines.

**C.** Fear on the part of the child to empty their bowels at nursery school, thus delaying bowel movements till returning home in the late afternoon.

**3.** Certain anal problems, such as anal sores, a congenitally narrowed anus, and congenital megacolon can cause constipation.

Most parents immediately resort to laxatives as soon as constipation occurs in their children, unaware that these have many side effects and only bring short-term relief. Pediatric constipation is highly responsive to Chinese infant massage which has no side effects.

# Patterns & Their Treatment

## Replete heat pattern (*shi re xing*)

**Disease causes:** This may be due either to overeating rich, greasy foods, overeating in general, or irregular bathroom habits in an otherwise replete or robust child.

**Main signs & symptoms:** Constipation or lack of bowel movement for several days in an otherwise healthy robust child or constipation in a child with heat signs, such as flushed face, red lips, excessive body heat or fever, bad breath, excessive thirst with a desire for cold drinks, a full feeling and stuffiness in the chest and abdomen, poor appetite, abdominal distention and pain, and scanty, dark urine

**Treatment principles:** Clear heat from the stomach and intestines and disinhibit the bowels

**Treatment methods:**

**1.** Rub the line on the lateral palmar edge of the index finger, pushing in one direction only from the base of the index finger to the tip 100-300 times. (Fig. 109) This is called slightly draining the Large Intestine Channel. Stimulation of this point in this manner clears heat and drains repletion from the large intestine.

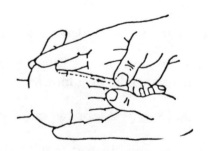

**Figure 109**

2. Rub the circle on the palm of the hand 100-300 times. This circle's center is the center of the palm and its radius is 2/3 the length from the center of the palm to the transverse crease at the base of the middle finger. (Fig. 110) This is called moving or transporting the Eight Trigrams. Stimulation of this point in this manner moves and quickens the qi and blood and harmonizes the five major organs.

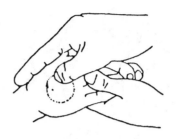

**Figure 110**

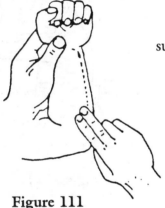

3. Rub the line on the medial (*i.e.*, ulnar), anterior surface of the forearm, pushing in one direction only from the elbow to the wrist in that direction only 100-300 times. (Fig. 111) This is called straight pushing the Six Bowels. Stimulation of this point clears heat, cools the blood, and resolves toxins.

**Figure 111**

4. Press and knead the point on the back side of the forearm directly above or proximal to the center of the back of the wrist 100-300 times. (Fig. 112) This point is called *Bo Yang Chi* (Arm Yang Pond). It corresponds to acupuncture point *Zhi Gou* (TH 6) in adults. This manipulation is called pressing and kneading Arm Yang Pond. Stimulation of this point in this manner opens the bowels.

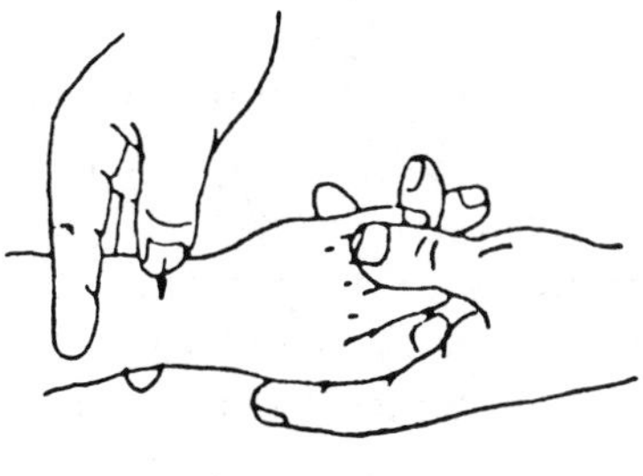

**Figure 112**

75

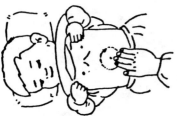

5. Round rub the abdomen around the navel clockwise with the hollow of the palm 100-500 times. (Fig. 113) This is called round rubbing the Abdomen. Stimulation of this point in this manner promotes digestion and bowel movements.

**Figure 113**

6. Rub both flanks or lateral costal regions simultaneously with the palms, pushing from underneath the armpits down to the level of the navel. (Fig. 114) This point is called *Xie Lei* (Flanks & Ribs). This maneuver is called rubbing the Flanks & Ribs. Stimulation of this point rectifies the qi (*i.e.*, downbears turbidity) and disperses masses in the abdomen.

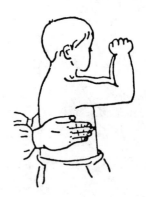

**Figure 114**

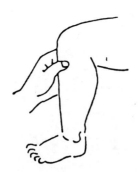

7. Knead the point below the knee on the lateral side of the lower legs between the tibia and fibula 50-100 times on both legs. (Fig. 115) This is called kneading Three *Li*. Stimulating this point harmonizes the stomach and intestines and promotes digestion.

**Figure 115**

8. Rub the line on the center of the sacrum, pushing from the small of the back downward to the tailbone 100-300 times. (Fig. 116) This is called pushing the Sacrum. Stimulating this point in this manner promotes bowel movements.

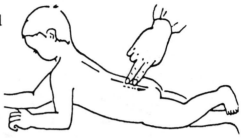

**Figure 116**

## Vacuity weakness pattern (*xu ruo xing*)

**Disease causes:** Constitutional weakness, chronic disease, or prolonged eating of raw, chilled, cold, and frozen foods and drinks

**Main signs & symptoms:** loose stools even though defecation is difficult, a pale complexion, light colored fingernails, loss of weight or a thin body, lack of energy

**Treatment principles:** Supplement the spleen and strengthen the center, harmonize the stomach and intestines and promote bowel movements

**Treatment methods:**

1. Slightly extend the child's thumb and rub the line on the lateral palmar edge of the thumb, pushing in one direction only from the tip to the base of the thumb 100-500 times. (Fig. 117) This is called supplementing the Spleen Channel. Stimulation of this point in this manner strengthens the spleen and supplements the center, thus strengthening digestion.

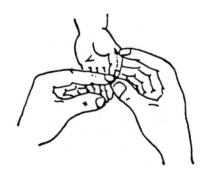

**Figure 117**

77

2. Rub the line on the lateral palmar side of the index finger, pushing from the base of the index finger to the tip 100-300 times. (Fig. 118) This is called slightly draining the Large Intestine Channel. Stimulation of this point in this manner drains repletion from the large intestine and promotes bowel movements.

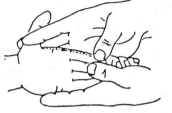

**Figure 118**

3. Knead the point in the depression between the two knuckles at the base of the ring and little fingers on the back side of the hand 100-300 times. (Fig. 119) This point is called *Shang Ma* (Upper Horse) and this maneuver is called kneading Upper Horse. Stimulation of this point enriches kidney yin and fortifies kidney yang.

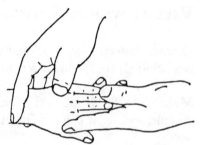

**Figure 119**

4. Press and knead the point on the back side of the forearm directly above or proximal to the center of the back of the wrist 100-300 times. (Fig. 120) This is called pressing Arm Yang Pond. Stimulation of this point in this manner opens the bowels.

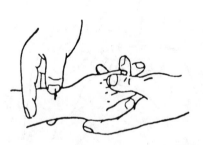

**Figure 120**

5. Rub the line on the middle of the anterior surface of the forearm, pushing from the wrist to the elbow 100-300 times. (Fig. 121) This is called pushing the Milky Way. Stimulation of this point clears heat and drains fire.

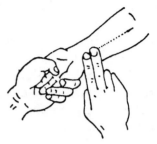

**Figure 121**

6. Round rub the abdomen around the navel clockwise with the hollow of the palm 100-500 times. (Fig. 122) This is called round rubbing the Abdomen. Stimulating this point in this manner promotes digestion and bowel movements.

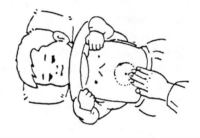

**Figure 122**

7. Knead the point below the knee on the lateral side of the lower leg between the tibia and fibula 50-100 times on both legs. (Fig. 123) This is called kneading Three *Li*. Stimulation of this point harmonizes the stomach and intestines and promotes digestion.

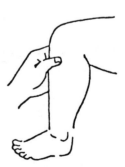

**Figure 123**

8. Rub the line on the middle of the sacrum, pushing in one direction only from the small of the back downward to the tailbone 100-300 times. (Fig. 124) This is called pushing the Sacrum. Stimulation of this point in this manner promotes bowel movements.

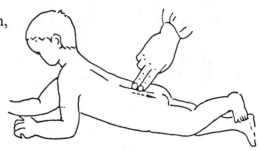

**Figure 124**

## Points for Special Attention

**1.** If an anal disease exists, it should first be treated by a physician. Once that disease is cured, the constipation will automatically be alleviated.

**2.** Constipation caused by improper feeding can be cured quickly by changing the baby's diet combined with pediatric *tui na*. Children fed cow's milk or milk powder are frequently constipated. In such cases, some fruit juice and honey should be introduced into their diets.

**3.** Children who are constipated should be fed more cooked vegetables and they should also drink more water. However, this should be warm water. It should not be cold water out of the tap or refrigerator.

**4.** Children should be well trained in good bowel habits. They should be encouraged to have bowel movements at regular times.

**5.** The above massage protocols should be performed once per day. Typically, the child will recover after 1-3 treatments.

# Excessive Drooling

During infancy, a certain amount of drooling is normal and natural. However, during teething, drooling and slobbering may become excessive. In that case, such excessive drooling will disappear as the teeth grow in. If the child continues to slobber excessively and unceasingly, this is called hypersalivation.

## Patterns & Their Treatment

### Food damage pattern (*shang shi xing*)

**Disease causes:** Overfeeding or feeding hard to digest foods

**Main signs & symptoms:** Excessive drooling accompanied by bad breath, red lips and tongue, abdominal distention, constipation, and dark, scanty urine

**Treatment principles:** Eliminate food stagnation and transform accumulations, clear heat and descend counterflow

**Treatment methods:** 1. Slightly bend the child's thumb and rub the line on the lateral palmar edge of the thumb, pushing in one direction only from the tip of the thumb to the base 100-500 times. This is called supplementing the Spleen Channel. (Fig. 125) Stimulation of this point strengthens the spleen and supplements the center, thus promoting digestion.

**Figure 125**

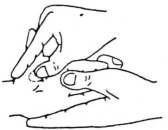

**Figure 126**

2. Knead the thenar eminence or major bulge at the base of the thumb 100-300 times. (Fig. 126) This is called kneading the Shuttered Gate. Stimulation of this point promotes digestion and removes accumulated food.

3. Rub the circle on the palm 100-300 times. This circle's center is the center of the palm and its radius is 2/3 the length from the center of the palm to the transverse crease at the base of the middle finger. (Fig. 127) This is called moving or transporting the Eight Trigrams. Stimulation of this point in this manner rectifies and frees the flow of qi and blood and harmonizes the five major organs.

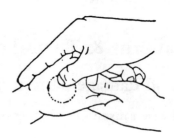

**Figure 127**

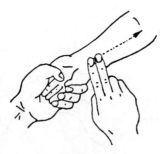

**Figure 128**

4. Rub the line on the middle of the anterior surface of the forearm, pushing in one direction only from the wrist to the elbow 100-300 times. (Fig. 128) This is called pushing the Milky Way. Stimulation of this point clears heat and drains fire.

5. Round rub the abdomen around the navel clockwise with the hollow of the palm 100-500 times. (Fig. 129) This is called round rubbing the Abdomen. Stimulation of this point in this manner promotes digestion and bowel movements.

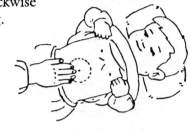

**Figure 129**

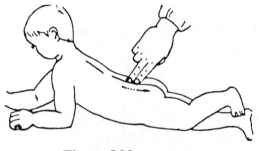

**Figure 130**

6. Rub the line on the center of the sacrum, pushing in one direction only from the small of the back downward to the tailbone 100-300 times. (Fig. 130) This is called pushing the Sacrum. Stimulation of this point in this manner promotes bowel movements and digestion.

## Vacuity weakness pattern (*xu ruo xing*)

**Disease causes:** Constitutional weakness, chronic disease, or prolonged consumption of raw and chilled, cold, or frozen foods and drinks

**Main signs & symptoms:** Excessive saliva which is clear and without smell, a sallow complexion, loss of weight or thin body, pale lips and tongue, cold limbs, and watery stool

**Treatment principles:** Supplement the spleen and harmonize the stomach

**Treatment methods:** 1. Slightly bend the child's thumb and rub the line on the lateral palmar edge of the thumb, pushing in one direction only from the tip to the base of the thumb 100-500 times. (See Fig. 125 above) This is called supplementing the Spleen Channel.

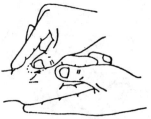

**Figure 131**

2. Knead the thenar eminence or major bulge at the base of the thumb 100-300 times. (Fig. 131) This is called kneading the Shuttered Gate. Stimulation of this point promotes digestion and removes accumulated food.

3. Rub the circle on the palm of the hand 100-300 times. This circle's center is the center of the palm and its radius is 2/3 the length of the center of the palm to the transverse crease at the base of the middle finger. (Fig. 132) This is called moving or transporting the Eight Trigrams. Stimulation of this point in this manner rectifies and frees the flow of qi and blood and harmonizes the functions of the five major organs.

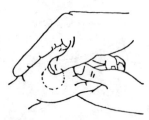

**Figure 132**

4. Rub the line on the lateral anterior surface of the forearm, pushing in one direction only from the wrist to the elbow 100-300 times. (Fig. 133) This is called pushing the Three Gates. Stimulating this point supplements the qi and fortifies yang.

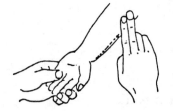

**Figure 133**

5. Round rub the abdomen around the navel counterclockwise with the hollow of the palm 100-500 times. (See Fig. 129 above) This is called round rubbing the Abdomen. Stimulating this point in this manner strengthens the digestion.

6. First apply some massage medium to the child's back. Then massage along the center of the spine from above to below 3 times. Next, put both hands on either side of the tailbone. Grasp and lift the skin with the thumbs and index and middle fingers of both hands, rolling up the skin from the tailbone to the base of the neck 3-5 times. (Fig. 134) This is called pinching and pulling the Spine. Stimulation of this point in this manner strengthens the constitution and supports the righteous qi.

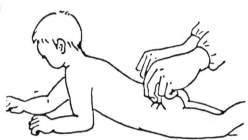

**Figure 134**

## Points for Special Attention

**1.** Some diseases of the nervous system can cause excessive salivation, such as facial nerve paralysis. In such cases, emphasis should be on treating the primary or causative disease.

**2.** If excessive slobbering occurs suddenly, check for inflammation or stimulation of the lining of the mouth by a foreign object. The child may have eaten something irritating. If so, remove this immediately.

**3.** Saliva flowing from the mouth may wet the clothes and dampen the skin causing skin inflammation or eczema. In cases of excessive salivation, the skin should be kept as clean and dry as possible.

**4.** The above massage protocols are performed once per day. Typically the child will recover after 1-3 treatments.

# Common Cold

The common cold is the most common disease of childhood. It is caused by unsuitable clothing, changes in the weather, or infection. It may occur in any season, but it is most common in winter and spring. Its main symptoms are fever, chills, stuffy nose, nasal discharge, cough, headache, and general aching. The protocols given below are for the treatment of a mild cold without prominent fever or cough. If a cold is accompanied by either fever or a cough, one should treat those symptoms. Both fever and cough are discussed in following chapters.

## Patterns & Their Treatment

### Wind cold pattern (*feng han xing*)

**Disease causes:** These have been discussed above.

**Main signs & symptoms:** Severe chills, slight fever, no sweating, stuffy nose, sniffling, clear nasal mucus, sneezing, itching of the throat, headache

**Treatment principles:** Relieve the exterior, expel wind, and disperse cold

**Treatment methods:**

1. Rub the line on the palmar surface of the terminal phalange of the ring finger, pushing in one direction only from the fingertip to the transverse crease of the

second knuckle 100-500 times. (Fig. 135)
This point is called *Fei Jing* (Lung
Channel) and this maneuver is called
supplementing the Lung Channel.
Stimulating this point in
this manner replenishes and
restores the lung qi while
expelling wind
and scattering cold.

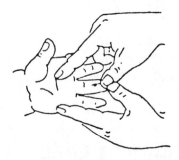

**Figure 135**

2. Nip and knead the two points in the depressions on
both sides of the knuckle at the base of the
middle finger on the back of
the hand. Nip 3-5 times and knead 100-300
times. (Fig. 136) These points are
called *Er Shan Men* (Two Flapping Gates).
This maneuver is called nipping and kneading
the Two Flapping Gates. Stimulation of
these points relieves or resolves the
exterior by promoting sweating. It also
promotes the free flow of qi and blood
and relaxes the muscles and tendons.

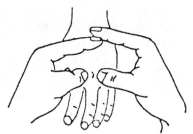

**Figure 136**

3. Rub the line on the lateral anterior
surface of the forearm, pushing in one
direction only from the wrist
to the elbow. (Fig. 137) This is called
pushing the Three Gates. Stimulation of
this point supplements the qi and
fortifies yang, disperses cold
and relieves the exterior.

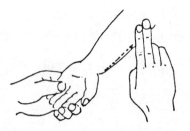

**Figure 137**

4. Rub the midline of the forehead, pushing
thumb over thumb alternately beginning
at the midpoint between the eyebrows
up to the anterior hairline 50-100 times.
Push in one direction only. (Fig. 138)
This point is called *Tian Men*
(Heavenly Gate) and this maneuver
is called opening Heaven's Gate.
Stimulation of this point dispels
pathogenic wind from the exterior
of the body and stops headache.

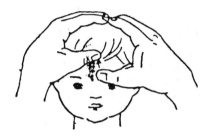

**Figure 138**

5. Push apart the forehead using the thumbs of both
hands 50-100 times. Push in one direction only from the
midline of the forehead to the temples. (Fig. 139) This
point is called *Kan Gong* (Water Palace)
and this manipulation is called pushing
apart the Water Palace. Stimulation of
this point induces sweating and dispels
pathogens from the exterior.
It also relieves headache.

**Figure 139**

6. Knead the temples lateral to the outer edges of
the eyebrows in the depression in front of the
hairline 50-100 times. (Fig. 140) This
point is called *Tai Yang* (Supreme Yang,
*i.e.*, the sun). This maneuver is called
kneading Supreme Yang. Stimulation of this
point dispels pathogenic wind from
the exterior and relieves headache.

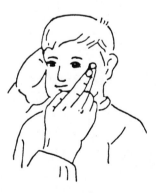

**Figure 140**

7. Knead the points lateral to or on the outside of the edges of the nostrils. Then lightly knead both nostril themselves 50-100 times. (Fig. 141) This point is called *Huang Feng Ru Dong* (Wasp Entering a Cave). This manipulation is, therefore, called kneading the Wasp Entering the Cave. Stimulation of this point induces sweating thus dispelling pathogens from the exterior of the body as well as opening the nasal passages and relieving stuffiness and sneezing.

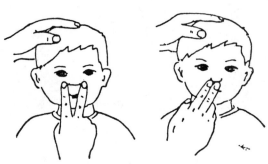

**Figure 141**

8. Rub the line on the back of the neck, pushing in one direction only from the hairline to the bulging bone (C7) at the base of the neck 100-500 times. (Fig. 142) This is called pushing the Heavenly Pillar Bones. Stimulation of this point promotes descension of the qi and relieves the exterior by means of diaphoresis.

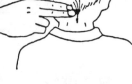

**Figure 142**

# Wind heat pattern (*feng re xing*)

**Disease causes:** These have been discussed above.

**Main signs & symptoms:** Mild chilliness, sweating, stuffy nose, sniffling, thick yellow nasal mucus, sneezing, sore throat, dry mouth, thirst, headache

**Treatment principles:** Relieve the exterior, expel wind, and clear heat

**Treatment methods:**

1. Rub the line on the center of the palmar surface of the last phalange of the ring finger, pushing in one direction only from the transverse crease of the second knuckle to the tip of the ring finger 100-500 times. (Fig. 143) This is called draining the Lung Channel. Stimulation of this point in this way clears heat from the lungs.

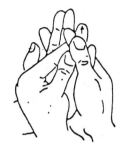

**Figure 143**

2. Rub the circle on the palm of the hand 100-300 times. This circle's center is the center of the palm and its radius is 2/3 the length from the center of the palm to the transverse crease at the base of the middle finger. (Fig. 144) This is called moving or transporting the Eight Trigrams. Stimulation of this point moves and quickens the flow of qi and blood as well as harmonizes the functions of the five major organs.

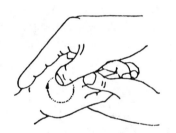

**Figure 144**

3. Rub the line on the midline of the anterior surface of the forearm, pushing in one direction only from the wrist to the elbow 100-300 times. (Fig. 145) This is called pushing the Milky Way. Stimulation of this point clears pathogenic heat and relieves the exterior.

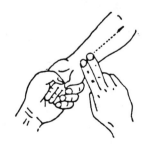

**Figure 145**

91

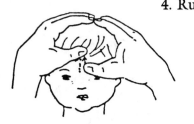

**Figure 146**

4. Rub the line on the midline of the forehead, pushing in one direction only thumb over thumb alternately from the midpoint of the eyebrows to the anterior hairline 50-100 times. (Fig. 146) This is called opening the Heavenly Gate. Stimulation of this point dispels pathogenic wind from the body and relieves headache.

5. Push apart the forehead with both thumbs, pushing in one direction only from the center of the forehead to the temples 50-100 times. (Fig. 147) This is called pushing apart the Water Palace and stimulation of this point dispels pathogens from the exterior and relieves headache.

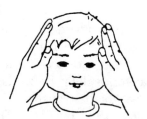

**Figure 147**

6. Knead the temples with the fingertips of the middle fingers of both hands simultaneously. Knead 50-100 times in the depression behind the outside tip of the eyebrows and the anterior hairline. (Fig. 148) This is called kneading Supreme Yang. Stimulation of this point dispels pathogenic wind from the exterior and relieves headache.

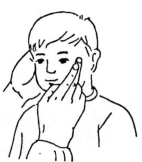

**Figure 148**

7. Knead the points lateral to the outside edges of the nostril and then lightly knead the nostrils themselves 50-100 times. (Fig. 149) This is called kneading the Wasp Entering the Cave. Stimulation of this point relieves the exterior and also disinhibits the nose, treating nasal congestion and sneezing.

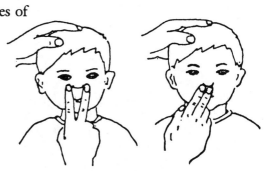

**Figure 149**

8. Rub the line on the back of the neck, pushing from the hairline to the bulging bone (C7) at the base of the neck 100-500 times. (Fig. 150) This is called pushing the Heavenly Pillar Bones. Stimulation of this point downbears lung qi and relieves the exterior by means of diaphoresis.

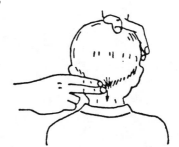

**Figure 150**

## Points for Special Attention

**1.** Be sure the child drinks plenty of water.

**2.** Do not overdress the child during warm weather. Overdressing easily induces sweating, thus increasing the likelihood of catching cold.

**3.** These massage protocols can be performed once per day in light cases and twice per day in serious cases. Typically, the child will recover after 1-3 treatments.

CHAPTER
8

# Cough

Cough in children is the most common respiratory pediatric complaint. It is most common in winter and spring, but it may occur in any season. Cough as a symptom may be associated with any of a number of respiratory tract diseases. These include the common cold, bronchitis, asthma, and pneumonia. If cough is the single most important symptom, other symptoms being mild or nonexistent, cough is generally diagnosed as being due to bronchitis. Bronchitis is then further divided into acute and chronic types.

The diagnosis of bronchitis in a child usually causes much anxiety in the parents who may then rush out and try all kinds of medicines. These may or may not be effective and they may even sometimes prolong the cough or result in increased risk of frequent relapse. Chinese pediatric *tui na* is a simple yet effective method of treating either acute or chronic cough in children without side effects. Typically, Chinese infant massage can quickly cure most coughs.

## Patterns & Their Treatments

### Wind cold pattern (*feng han xing*)

**Disease causes:** The same as wind cold common cold discussed above.

**Main signs & symptoms:** Cough with thin white or clear mucus, stuffy nose, a watery, white nasal discharge, severe chills, slight fever, no sweating, and headache

**Treatment principles:** Relieve the exterior, expel wind, and disperse cold

**Treatment methods:**

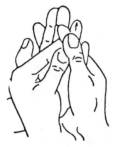

Figure 151

1. Rub the line on the palmar surface of the tip of the ring finger, pushing in one direction only from the transverse crease of the second knuckle toward the tip 100-500 times. (Fig. 151) This is called slightly draining the Lung Channel. Stimulation of this point in this manner drains pathogens from the lungs.

2. Rub the circle on the palm of the hand 100-300 times. This circle's center is the center of the palm and its radius is 2/3 the length from the center to the transverse crease at the base of the middle finger. (Fig. 152) This is called moving or transporting the Eight Trigrams. Stimulation of this point in this manner rectifies and frees the flow of qi and blood as well as harmonizes the functions of the five major organs.

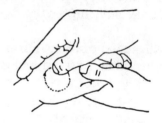

Figure 152

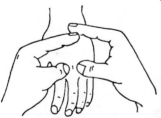

Figure 153

3. Nip and knead the two points in the depression just proximal or above the knuckle at the base of the middle finger on the back of the hand. Nip 3-5 times and knead 100-300 times. (Fig. 153) This is called nipping and kneading the Two Flapping Gates. Stimulation of this point relieves the exterior and promotes sweating, frees the flow of qi and blood, and relaxes the muscles and tendons.

4. Rub the line on the lateral anterior surface of the forearm, pushing in one direction only from the wrist to the elbow 100-300 times. (Fig. 154) This is called pushing the Three Gates. Stimulation of this point warms yang and disperses cold.

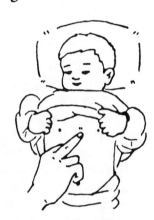

**Figure 154**

5. With both thumbs, push apart the horizontal line connecting the nipples from the midpoint of this line to both breasts 100-500 times. Then knead the midpoint 100-300 times. (Fig. 155) This point is called *Shan Zhong* (Central Altar). It corresponds to acupuncture point CV 17. Stimulation of this point rectifies the qi of the lungs and stops coughing.

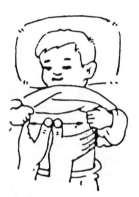

**Figure 155**

6. Knead the points just lateral and just below both nipples with the index and middle fingers of both hands 100-300 times. (Fig. 156) The points just lateral to the nipples are called *Ru Pang* (Side of the Breast) and the points just below the nipples are called *Ru Gen* (Breast Root). Stimulation of these points soothes chest oppression, rectifies the qi, relieves cough, and transforms phlegm.

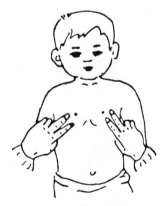

**Figure 156**

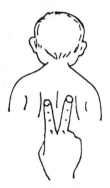

**Figure 157**

7. Knead the points located 1/2 the distance between the center of the spine and the inside edge of the scapula or shoulder blades just lateral to the lower border to the spinous process of the 3rd thoracic vertebra (T3) 50-100 times. Knead these points with the index and middle fingers simultaneously. (Fig. 158). This point is called *Fei Shu* (Lung Transport). Stimulating this point in this manner rectifies the qi of the lungs and stops coughing.

8. Push apart the curves along the medial border of both shoulder blades, pushing in one direction only from above to below with the pads of the thumbs 100-300 times. (Fig. 158) This is called pushing apart Lung Transport. Stimulation of this point in this manner relieves chest oppression, rectifies the qi of the lungs, transforms phlegm, and stops coughing.

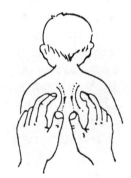

**Figure 158**

9. Rub the line in the center of the back of the neck, pushing in one direction only from the hairline to the bulging bone (C7) at the base of the neck 100-500 times. (Fig. 159) This is called pushing the Heavenly Pillar Bones. Stimulation of this point promotes the descension of qi and thus helps stop coughing.

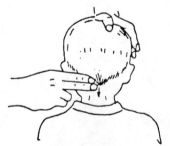

**Figure 159**

# Wind heat pattern (*feng re xing*)

**Disease causes:** Discussed above under common cold

**Main signs & symptoms:** Cough with thick, yellow mucus, a stuffy nose with thick, yellow nasal discharge, slight chills, higher fever, slight sweating, thirst, sore throat, and headache

**Treatment principles:** Relieve the exterior, expel wind, and clear heat

**Treatment methods:**

1. Rub the line on the pad of the ring finger, pushing in one direction only from the transverse crease of the second knuckle to the tip 100-500 times. (Fig. 160) This is called slightly draining the Lung Channel. Stimulation of this point in this manner drains pathogens from the lungs.

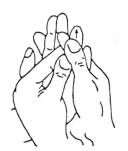

**Figure 160**

2. Rub the circle on the palm of the hand 100-300 times. This circle's center is the center of the palm and its radius is 2/3 the length from the center of the palm to the transverse crease at the base of the middle finger. (Fig. 161) This is called moving or transporting the Eight Trigrams. Stimulation of this point in this manner rectifies and frees the flow of the qi and blood and harmonizes the functions of the five major organs.

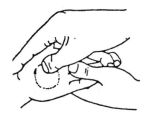

**Figure 161**

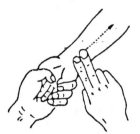

**Figure 162**

3. Rub the line on the center of the anterior surface of the forearm, pushing in one direction only from the wrist to the elbow 100-300 times. (Fig. 162) This is called pushing the Milky Way. It clears heat and relieves the exterior as well as drains pathogenic fire.

4. With both thumbs, push apart the line joining the nipples, pushing from the midline toward the breasts in one direction only 100-500 times. Then knead the midpoint of this line 100-300 times. (Fig. 163) This is called pushing apart and kneading the Central Altar. Stimulation of this point rectifies the qi of the lungs and stops coughing.

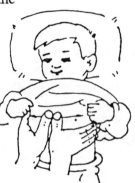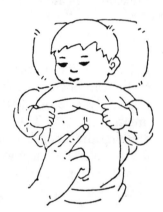

**Figure 163**

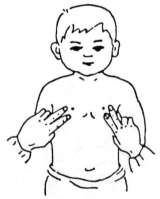

**Figure 164**

5. Knead the points just lateral and just below both nipples with the index and middle fingers of both hands 100-300 times. (Fig. 164) This is called kneading the Sides of the Breasts and Breast Root. Stimulation of these points soothes chest oppression, rectifies the qi, relieves cough, and transforms phlegm.

6. Knead the points located 1/2 the distance between
the center of the spine and the inside edge
of the shoulder blades lateral to the lower
border of the spinous process of the 3rd
thoracic vertebra (T3) with index and
middle fingers simultaneously 50-100 times.
(Fig. 165) This is called kneading Lung
Transport. Stimulation of this point in
this manner rectifies the lung
qi and stops coughing.

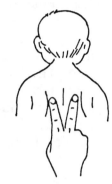

**Figure 165**

7. With both thumbs, push apart the curves along the
medial or inner border of the shoulder blades,
pushing in one direction only from above to
below 100-300 times. (Fig. 166) This is
called pushing apart Lung Transport.
Stimulation of this point in this manner
relieves chest oppression, rectifies
the qi of the lungs, transforms phlegm,
and stops coughing.

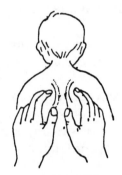

**Figure 166**

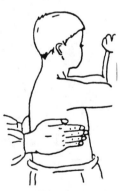

**Figure 167**

8. Rub the lateral costal regions with both palms,
pushing from underneath the armpits down
to the level of the navel in one direction
only 100-300 times. (Fig. 169) This is
called pushing the Flanks & Ribs.
Stimulation of this point
rectifies the qi and
transforms phlegm.

9. Rub the line on the center of the back of the neck, pushing in one direction only downward from the hairline to the bulging bone (C7) at the base of the neck 100-500 times. (Fig. 168) This is called pushing the Heavenly Pillar Bones. Stimulation of this point promotes the downward descension of the qi and thus helps stop coughing and relieves the exterior through diaphoresis.

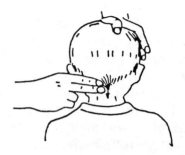

**Figure 168**

## Vacuity weakness pattern (*xu ruo xing*)

**Disease causes:** Constitutional weakness, prolonged disease, or prolonged cough due to mistreatment or lack of treatment.

**Main signs & symptoms:** Prolonged cough, either an unproductive cough with little mucus or a productive cough with a lot of mucus, slight fever, a pale face, spontaneous sweating or night sweating, poor appetite, listlessness and fatigue, and weight loss or thinness

**Treatment principles:** Supplement the lungs and spleen, descend the qi, and stop coughing

**Treatment methods:**

1. Rub the line on the palmar surface of the ring finger tip, pushing in one direction only from the tip to the transverse crease of the third knuckle 100-500 times. (Fig. 169) This is called supplementing the Lung Channel. Stimulation of this point in this manner replenishes and restores the lung qi.

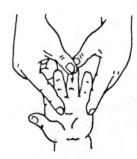

**Figure 169**

2. Slightly bend the child's thumb and rub the line on the lateral palmar edge of the thumb, pushing in one direction only from the tip to the base of the thumb 100-500 times. (Fig. 170) This is called supplementing the Spleen Channel. Stimulation of this point in this manner strengthens the spleen and supplements the center, thus strengthening the root of qi and blood production.

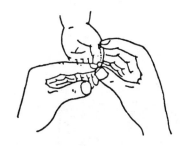

**Figure 170**

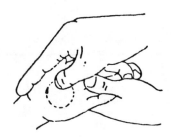

**Figure 171**

3. Rub the circle on the palm of the hand 100-300 times. This circle's center is the center of the palm and its radius is 2/3 the length from the center of the palm to the transverse crease at the base of the middle finger. (Fig. 171) This is called moving or transporting the Eight Trigrams. Stimulation of this point rectifies and frees the flow of qi and blood as well as harmonizes the functions of the five major organs.

4. With the tips of the thumbs, push apart the line joining the nipples, pushing from the midpoint to the breasts in one direction only 100-500 times. Then knead the midpoint 100-300 times. (Fig. 172) This is called pushing apart and kneading the Central Altar. Stimulation of this point in this manner rectifies the qi of the lungs and stops coughing.

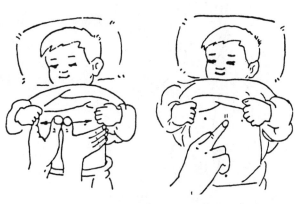

**Figure 172**

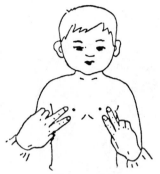

**Figure 173**

5. Knead the points just lateral and just below the nipples with the index and middle fingers of both hands 100-300 times. (Fig. 173) This is called kneading the sides of the Breast and Breast Root. Stimulation of these points soothes chest oppression, rectifies the qi, relieves cough, and transforms phlegm.

6. Knead the point above the navel in the middle of the upper abdomen with the hollow of the palm clockwise 100-300 times. (Fig. 174) This is called kneading the Central Venter. Stimulation of this point in this manner strengthens the spleen and stomach, thus strengthening the digestion, the source of production of the qi and blood.

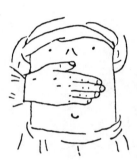

**Figure 174**

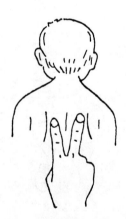

**Figure 175**

7. Knead the points located 1/2 way between the center of the spine and the inside edge of the scapula lateral to the lower edge of the spinous process of the 3rd thoracic vertebra (T3) with the index and middle fingers simultaneously 50-100 times. (Fig. 175) This is called kneading Lung Transport. Stimulation of this point in this manner rectifies the qi of the lungs and stops coughing.

8. With the tips of both thumbs, push apart the curves on the inner borders of both shoulder blades, pushing in one direction only from above to below 100-300 times. (Fig. 176) This is called pushing apart Lung Transport. Stimulation of this point in this manner rectifies the qi of the lungs and stops coughing.

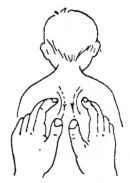

**Figure 176**

9. First apply some massage medium to the child's back and massage lightly along the center of the spine from above to below 3 times. Then place the hands on each side of the tailbone. Grasp and lift the skin with the thumbs and middle and index fingers, rolling the skin upward from the tailbone to the base of the neck 3-5 times. (Fig. 177) This is called pinching and pulling the Spine. Stimulation of this point strengthens the constitution and supports the righteous qi.

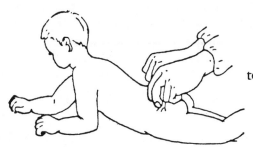

**Figure 177**

## Points for Special Attention

1. Cough with fever may have a number of causes. Therefore, when cough is accompanied by fever, it is first necessary to identify its diagnosis and then to treat it according to its cause. One should not use cough-suppressing medication indiscriminately since it may hamper the expectoration of phlegm and thus retard the healing process.

**2.** During a cough, fluid intake should be higher than usual. One can give water or fruit juice, especially pear juice, in cases with a dry, unproductive cough. However, greasy, oily foods should be avoided.

**3.** The air in the child's room should be kept fresh, and the child should neither be overdressed or underdressed.

**4.** When healthy, the child should be encouraged to exercise regularly. Exercise is important to enhance their resistance to disease.

**5.** Generally, the above protocols are performed once per day. However, they may be done twice per day in more serious cases. Typically, children will recover after 1-3 day's treatment.

For more information on the TCM diagnosis and treatment of pediatric bronchitis, the interested reader should see Xiao Shu-qin *et al.*'s *Pediatric Bronchitis: Its TCM Cause, Diagnosis, Treatment, & Prevention* also published by Blue Poppy Press.

CHAPTER

9

# Fever

Fever is another common symptom of childhood diseases. When a child has a fever, he or she will manifest this in several different ways. They may cry, fidget restlessly, or may become listless. Usually their urine and stool are abnormal. They may also have a cough and/or poor appetite. If any of these symptoms are observed, the parent should feel the child's head or take their temperature to determine whether or not there is a fever.

There are many causes for fever, such as a common cold or flu, some other infectious disease, or a low grade fever due to some functional abnormality. However, most commonly, pediatric fevers are associated with the common cold. Below are treatment protocols for the treatment of fever due to a common cold and low fever due functional abnormality.

## Patterns & Their Treatment

### Wind cold pattern (*feng han xing*)

**Disease causes:** Discussed above under common cold

**Main signs & symptoms:** Low fever, severe chills, no sweating, stuffy nose, sniffling, clear nasal discharge, sneezing, itchy throat, and headache

**Treatment principles:** Relieve the exterior, expel wind, and disperse cold

**Treatment methods:**

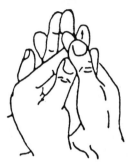

**Figure 178**

1. Rub the line on the palmar surface of the tip of the ring finger, pushing in one direction only from the transverse crease near the third knuckle to the tip 100-500 times. (Fig. 178) This is called slightly draining the Lung Channel. Stimulation of this point in this manner drains pathogenic qi from the lungs.

2. Nip and knead the two points in the depression just proximal to the first knuckle of the middle finger on the back of the hand. Nip 3-5 times and knead 100-300 times. (Fig. 179) This is called nipping and kneading the Two Flapping Gates. Stimulation of this point relieves the exterior, promotes sweating, frees the flow of qi and blood, and relaxes the muscles and tendons.

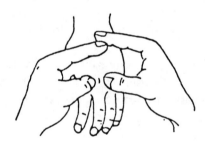

**Figure 179**

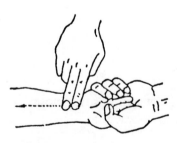

**Figure 180**

3. Rub the line in the middle of the anterior surface of the forearm, pushing in one direction only from the wrist to the elbow 100-300 times. (Fig. 180) This is called pushing the Milky Way. Stimulation of this point clears heat and relieves the exterior.

4. Rub the line on the middle of the forehead, pushing thumb over thumb upward from the midpoint between the eyebrows to the anterior hairline in one direction only 50-100 times. (Fig. 181) This is called opening the Heavenly Gate. Stimulation of this point relieves the exterior, dispels wind, and stops headache at the same time as it calms the spirit.

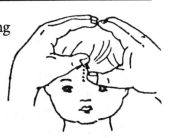

**Figure 181**

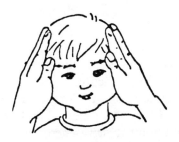

**Figure 182**

5. Push apart the line above the eyebrows, pushing with both thumbs from the midpoint to ends of the eyebrows 50-100 times. (Fig. 182) This is called pushing apart the Water Palace. Stimulation of this point relieves the exterior, dispels pathogens, and stops headache.

6. Knead the midpoint of the temples in the depression behind the lateral end of the eyebrows and in front of the anterior hairline 50-100 times. (Fig. 183) This is called kneading Supreme Yang. Stimulation of this point relieves the exterior, dispels wind, and stops pain.

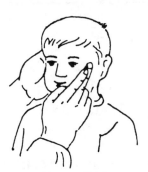

**Figure 183**

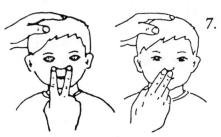

**Figure 184**

7. Knead the points just lateral to the outside edges of the nostrils and then lightly knead inside both nostrils 50-100 times. (Fig. 184) This is called Wasp Entering a Cave. Stimulation of this point promotes sweating and dispels pathogens from the exterior of the body at the same time as it frees the nasal passages.

8. Rub the line in the center of the back of the neck, pushing in one direction only downward from the hairline to the bulging bone (C7) at the base of the neck 100-500 times. (Fig. 185) This is called pushing the Heavenly Pillar Bones. Stimulation of this point promotes the downward descension of qi and relieves the exterior by inducing perspiration.

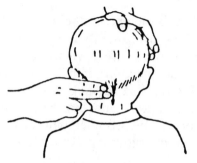

**Figure 185**

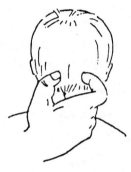

**Figure 186**

9. Press and grasp the two points just slightly above the posterior hairline and in the depression between the mastoid process and the long muscles at the back of the neck 5-10 times. (Fig. 186) This is the same point which in acupuncture is called *Feng Chi* (Wind Pond, GB 20). This manipulation is called pressing and grasping Wind Pond. Stimulation of this point relieves the exterior and dispels wind.

## Wind heat pattern (*feng re xing*)

**Disease causes:** Discussed above under common cold

**Main signs & symptoms:** High fever, slight chills, slight sweating, stuffy nose, sniffling, thick, yellow mucus, sneezing, sore throat, dry mouth, thirst, and headache

**Treatment principles:** Relieve the exterior, expel wind, and clear heat

**Treatment methods:**

1. Rub the line on the palmar surface of the tip of the ring finger, pushing in one direction only from the transverse crease of the third knuckle to the tip 100-500 times. (Fig. 187) This is called slightly draining the Lung Channel. Stimulation of this point in this manner drains pathogens from the lung.

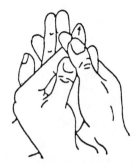

**Figure 187**

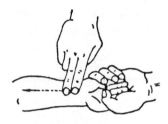

**Figure 188**

2. Rub the line in the center of the anterior surface of the forearm, pushing in one direction only from the wrist to the elbow 100-300 times. (Fig. 188) This is called pushing the Milky Way. Stimulation of this point clears heat and relieves the exterior.

3. Rub the line on the medial (*i.e.*, ulnar), anterior surface of the forearm, pushing in one direction only from the elbow to the wrist 100-300 times. (Fig. 189) This point is called *Liu Fu* (the Six Bowels). This manipulation is called pushing the Six Bowels. Stimulation of this point clears heat, cools the blood, and resolves toxins.

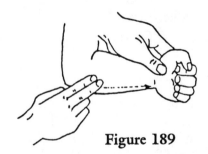

**Figure 189**

4. Rub the line on the center of the forehead, thumb over thumb from the mid-point of the eyebrows to the anterior hairline in one direction only 50-100 times. (Fig. 190 below) This is called opening Heaven's Gate. Stimulation of this point relieves the exterior, dispels wind, and stops headache.

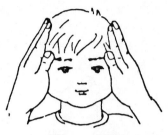

**Figure 190**

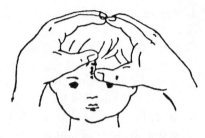

**Figure 191**

5. With the tips of the thumbs, push apart the line above the eyebrows, pushing in one direction only from the midpoint of the eyebrows out towards the ends of the eyebrows 50-100 times. (Fig. 191) This is called pushing apart the Water Palace. Stimulation of this point relieves the exterior, dispels wind, and stops headache.

6. Knead the points in the center of the temples lateral to the tips of the eyebrows and in front of the anterior hairline 50-100 times. (Fig. 192) This is called kneading Supreme Yang. Stimulation of this point relieves the exterior, dispels wind, and stops headache.

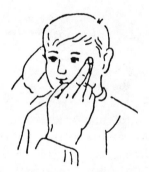

**Figure 192**

7. Knead the points just lateral to the outside edges of the nostrils and then lightly knead the nostrils themselves 50-100 times. (Fig. 193) This is called Wasp Entering a Cave. Stimulation of this point relieves the exterior, promotes sweating, and frees the flow of the nasal passages.

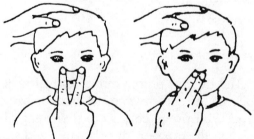

**Figure 193**

8. Rub the line in the center of the back of the neck, pushing in one direction only downward from the hairline to the bulging bone (C7) at the base of the neck 100-500 times. (See Fig. 185 above) This is called pushing the Heavenly Pillar Bones. Stimulation of this point promotes the downward descension of qi and relieves the exterior by inducing perspiration.

9. Rub the line on the center of the spine, pushing in one direction only from the bulging bone (C7) at the base of the neck downward to the tailbone 100-300 times. (Fig. 194) This is called pushing the Spine. Stimulation of this point in this manner clears pathogenic heat, discharges pathogenic fire, and opens the bowels.

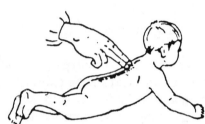

**Figure 194**

## Replete heat pattern (*shi re xing*)

**Disease causes:** This type of fever may be due to two main causes. First, it may be due to a common cold having progressed so that pathogens have invaded from the body's exterior to the interior. Secondly, overeating greasy, oily foods, overeating in general, and a replete constitution may result in the internal generation of heat.

**Main signs & symptoms:** High fever, flushed cheeks with red lips, a dry feeling in the mouth and nose, thirst with a desire to drink and a preference for cold drinks, shortness of breath, fidgeting, loss of appetite, constipation, and dark, scanty urine

**Treatment principles:** Clear heat, drain fire, and promote bowel movements

**Treatment methods:** 1. Rub the line on the palmar surface of the tip of the ring finger, pushing in one direction only from the transverse crease of the third knuckle to the tip 100-500 times. (Fig. 195 below) This is called slightly draining the Lung Channel. Stimulation of this point in this manner drains pathogens from the lungs.

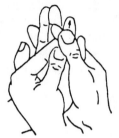

**Figure 195**

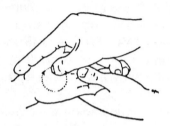

**Figure 196**

2. Rub the circle on the palm of the hand 100-300 times. This circle's center is the circle in the center of the palm and its radius is 2/3 the length from the center of the palm to the transverse crease at the base of the middle finger. (Fig. 196) This is called moving or transporting the Eight Trigrams. Stimulation of this point in this manner rectifies and frees the flow of qi and blood as well as harmonizes the functions of the five major organs.

3. Rub the line in the middle of the anterior surface of the forearm, pushing in one direction only from the wrist to the elbow 100-300 times. (Fig. 197) This is called pushing the Milky Way. Stimulation of this point clears heat and relieves the exterior.

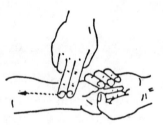

**Figure 197**

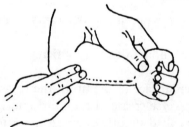

6. Rub the line on the medial (*i.e.*, ulnar), anterior surface of the forearm, pushing in one direction only from the elbow to the wrist 100-300 times. (Fig. 198) This is called pushing the Six Bowels. Stimulation of this point clears heat, cools the blood, and resolves toxins.

**Figure 198**

5. Round rub the abdomen around the navel clockwise with the hollow of the palm 100-500 times. (Fig. 199) This is called round rubbing the Abdomen. Stimulation of this point in this manner promotes digestion and bowel movements.

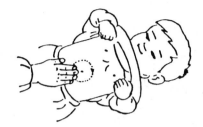

**Figure 199**

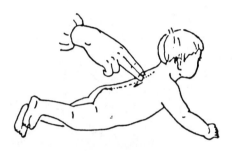

6. Rub the line on the center of the spine, pushing in one direction only downward from the bulging bone (C7) at the base of the neck to the tailbone 100-300 times. (Fig. 200) This is called pushing the Spine. Stimulation of this point in this manner clears pathogenic heat, discharges fire, and opens the bowels.

**Figure 200**

## Vacuity heat pattern (*xu re xing*)

**Disease causes:** This type of fever may be due to constitutional weakness, prolonged or chronic disease, or prolonged use of various medications. These may cause a functional disorder in the body's regulation of temperature.

**Main signs & symptoms:** Prolonged low grade fever, fever in the afternoon, a feverish sensation in the chest, palms of the hands, and soles of the feet, spontaneous sweating or night sweating, loss of weight or thinness, and poor appetite

**Treatment principles:** Enrich yin and clear heat

**Treatment methods:**

115

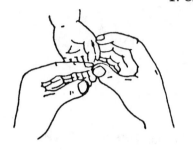

**Figure 201**

1. Slightly bend the child's thumb and rub the line on the lateral palmar edge of the thumb, pushing in one direction only from the tip of the thumb to its base 100-500 times. (Fig. 201) This is called supplementing the Spleen Channel. Stimulating this point in this manner strengthens the spleen and supplements the center, thus strengthening the source of the production of qi and blood.

2. Rub the line on the palmar surface of the tip of the ring finger, pushing in one direction only from the tip to the transverse crease of the third knuckle 100-500 times. (Fig. 202) This is called supplementing the Lung Channel. Stimulation of this point in this manner supplements the lungs.

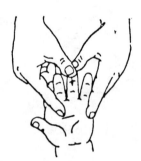

**Figure 202**

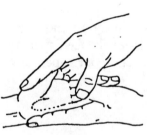

**Figure 203**

3. Rub the curve of the palm, pushing from the base of the little finger toward the base of the hand and thence upward toward the center of the palm 100-300 times. (Fig. 203) This point is called *Shui Di Lao Yue* (Fishing for the Moon in the Water). This method of manipulation is, therefore, called Fishing for the Moon in the Water. It is also called arc-pushing the Inner Palace of Labor. Stimulation of this point clears vacuity heat in the heart and kidney channels.

4. Knead the point in the depression just proximal to the knuckles at the base of the ring and little fingers on the back side of the hand 100-300 times. (Fig. 204) This point is called *Er Ren Shang Ma* (Two Men Upon a Horse). Therefore, this manipulation is called kneading Two Men Upon a Horse. Stimulation of this point enriches kidney yin and fortifies kidney yang.

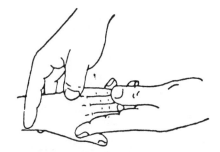

**Figure 204**

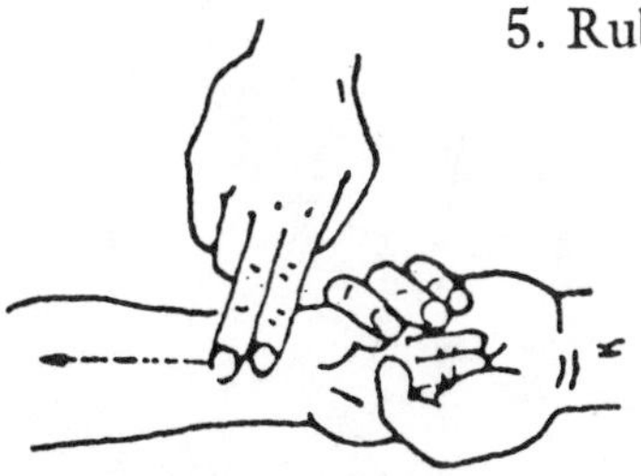

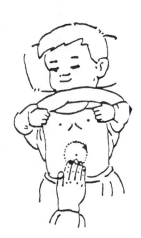

5. Rub the line in the middle of the anterior surface of the forearm, pushing in one direction only from the wrist to the elbow 100-300 times. (Fig. 205) This is called pushing the Milky Way. Stimulation of this point clears interior heat.

**Figure 205**

6. Round rub the abdomen around the navel clockwise with the hollow of the palm 100-500 times. (Fig. 206) This is called round rubbing the Abdomen. Stimulation of this point in this manner strengthens the spleen and supplements the center, thus promoting the source of production of the qi and blood and opening the bowels.

**Figure 206**

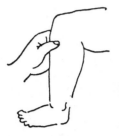

7. Knead the point below the knee on the lateral edge of the lower leg in between the tibia and fibula 50-100 times on both legs. (Fig. 207) This is called kneading three *Li*. Stimulation of this point harmonizes the stomach and intestines and promotes digestion.

**Figure 207**

8. Rub the line in the middle of the sole of the foot, pushing in one direction only from the ball of the foot to the base of the middle toes 100-300 times on both feet. (Fig. 208) This point is called *Yong Quan* (Bubbling Spring) and this maneuver is called pushing the Bubbling Spring. Stimulation of this point leads fire downward, thus reducing fever due to yin vacuity.

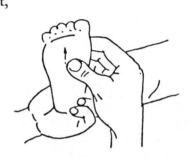

**Figure 208**

9. First apply some massage medium to the child's back and lightly massage the center of the spine from above to below 3 times. Then place the hands on either side of the tailbone. Grasp and lift the skin with the thumbs and index and middle fingers, rolling the skin upward from the tailbone to the base of the neck 3-5 times. (Fig. 209) This is called pinching and pulling the Spine. Stimulation of this point in this manner strengthens the constitution and supports the righteous qi.

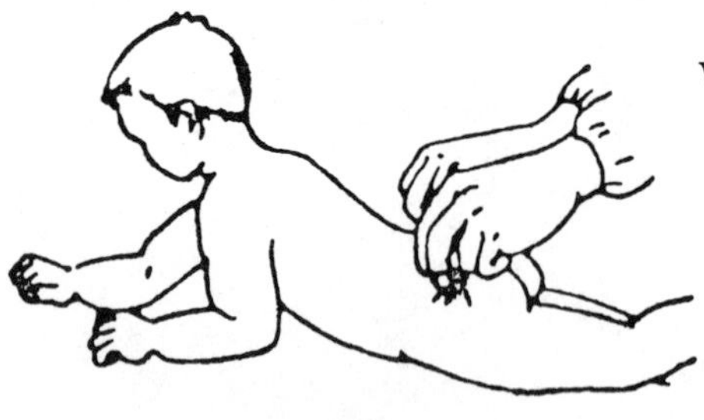

**Figure 209**

## Points for Special Attention

**1.** A child with fever should be nursed with the best of care. They should be sure to get proper rest and should drink plenty of water. In addition, they should be fed bland, easily digestible food and particularly more vegetables. The air in their room should be fresh and the room should be kept at an appropriate temperature.

**2.** There are many causes of fever. Antipyretics and antibiotics should be avoided unless diagnosis absolutely warrants their use. Steroids should especially be avoided. Such Western medicine may bring about temporary effect, but the risk of relapse is high. Overdoses of such medicinals are harmful, lowering resistance to disease and sensitivity of pathogens to them when their use is genuinely required. In addition, antibiotics and steroids should never be used for prolonged periods of time.

**3.** The above massage protocols can be performed once per day. However, in serious cases, they may be performed twice or even three times per day. Typically, most children will recover after 1-3 day's treatment.

CHAPTER
10

# Bedwetting

B edwetting or enuresis refers to involuntary urination in children over three years of age occurring most often during sleep at night. Some patients have this problem for years, continuing into later childhood. This causes them severe embarrassment and many may attempt to conceal their condition, thus developing emotional stress. In such cases after some time, they may become uncommunicative and moody.

In children under three years old, enuresis and bedwetting are not considered illnesses. In such young children, they are due to insufficient development of their cerebrospinal cord coupled with lack of forming good habits regarding the regular and timely voiding of urine.

**Main signs & symptoms:** Involuntary voiding of urine during sleep which occurs more commonly if the patient was fatigued during the day or on cloudy, rainy days. This may occur once every several nights in mild conditions but one, two, or more times per night in more severe conditions. If the disease becomes chronic, the patient may develop a sallow complexion, listlessness, fatigue, dizziness, soreness of the low back, spontaneous sweating, night sweating, and cold extremities.

**Treatment principles:** Supplement the kidneys and secure the essence

**Treatment methods:**

1. Slightly bend the child's thumb and rub the line on the lateral palmar edge of the thumb, pushing in one direction only from the tip to the base of the thumb

100-500 times. (Fig. 210) This is called supplementing the Spleen Channel. Stimulation of this point in this manner strengthens the spleen and supplements the center, thus promoting the source of production of the qi and blood.

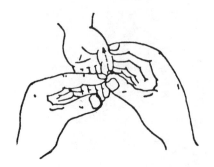

**Figure 210**

2. Rub the line on the medial palmar edge of the little finger and palm of the hand, pushing in one direction only from the base of the palm to the tip of the little finger 100-500 times. (Fig. 211) This point is called *Shen Jing* (the Kidney Channel). This maneuver is, therefore, called supplementing the Kidney Channel. Stimulation of this point supplements the kidneys and strengthens the body.

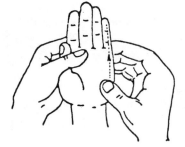

**Figure 211**

3. Rub the line on the palmar surface of the tip of the ring finger, pushing in one direction only from the tip to the transverse crease of the third knuckle 100-500 times. (Fig. 212) This is called supplementing the Lung Channel. Stimulation of this point in this manner supplements the lung qi.

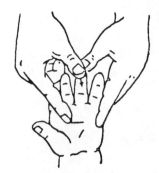

**Figure 212**

4. Knead the point in the depression just above or proximal to the first knuckles between the fourth and fifth fingers on the back side of the hand 100-300 times. (Fig. 213) This is called kneading Two Men Upon a Horse. Stimulation of this point enriches kidney yin and fortifies kidney yang.

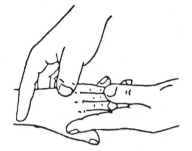

**Figure 213**

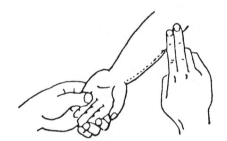

**Figure 214**

5. Knead the point in the center of the back of the hand 100-300 times. (Fig. 214) This is called kneading the Outer Palace of Labor. Stimulation of this point warms yang and disperses pathogenic cold. It especially warms the lower burner.

6. Rub the line on the lateral anterior surface of the forearm, pushing in one direction only from the wrist to the elbow 100-300 times. (Fig. 215) This is called pushing the Three Gates. Stimulation of this point supplements the qi and fortifies yang.

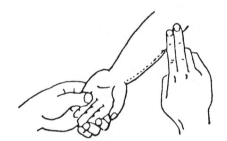

**Figure 215**

7. Press and knead the point at the midpoint of the line connecting the tips of both ears 100-300 times. (Fig. 216, next page) This point is called Hundred Convergences. It is the same as acupuncture point GV 20. this maneuvers is called kneading and pressing Hundred Convergences. Stimulation of this point in this manner calms the spirit and invigorates vital function, upbears yang and treats collapse.

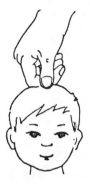

**Figure 216**

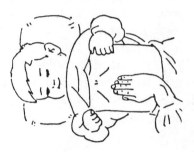

**Figure 217**

8. Knead the point at the midpoint of the lower abdomen 100-300 times. (Fig. 217) This point is called *Dan Tian* (Cinnabar Field). Therefore, this method of manipulation is called kneading the Cinnabar Field. Stimulation of this point supplements the kidneys.

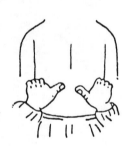

9. Knead the points on the lower back on either side of the lower border of the spinous process of the 2nd lumbar vertebra 100-200 times. (Fig. 218) This point is called *Shen Shu* (Kidney Transport). It is the same as acupuncture point Bl 23. This maneuver is called kneading Kidney Transport. Stimulation of this point supplements the kidneys.

**Figure 218**

10. Chafe the lower back by rubbing back and forth with the palm of the hand until the area feels warm. (Fig. 219) This is called chafing the Lower Back and stimulation of this point also warms and supplements the kidneys.

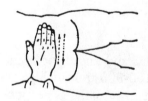

**Figure 219**

11. Knead the point on the posterior border of the tibia above the medial malleolus, *i.e.*, the inner ankle bone, 100-200 times on each leg. (Fig. 220) This point is called *San Yin Jiao* (Three Yin Intersection). It is the same as acupuncture point Sp 6. This maneuver is called kneading Three Yin Intersection and stimulation of this point in this manner supplements the kidneys and strengthens the spleen.

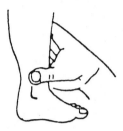

**Figure 220**

## Points for Special Attention

**1.** After the child's birth, the parents should pay attention in order to foster in the child good habits of personal hygiene. They can help foster such good habits in their son or daughter by always changing their diapers as soon as they are wet and training their children to develop regular urination habits.

**2.** Before the child goes to bed, the parents should avoid tiring, frightening, or exciting them.

**3.** The child should not be allowed to drink large amounts of fluids in the evening.

**4.** The parents should try to be patient in educating and training their children, thus dispelling their worries and fears. They should not reprimand their children wantonly.

**5.** This massage protocol can be performed once per day. Six such treatments equal one course of treatment. Typically, most children with this condition are cured after one course of treatment. If the child is not cured, they can be given another course after a 1-2 day rest.

**6.** When this protocol is performed by a professional practitioner in the clinic, one can moxa the last four points in this protocol, Cinnabar Field, Kidney Transport, the Lower Back, and Three Yin Intersection, in combination with their massage for better results.

# CHAPTER 11

# Night Crying

Night crying as a traditional Chinese disease category, along with abdominal pain, covers what is called colic in the West. In this case, the child appears normal during the day but cries during the night either intermittently or incessantly. Some children cry all night while others cry at only specific hours each night. Most often, this complaint occurs in children under six months of age. In older children, the cause is more often fright and is not associated with colic.

## Patterns & Their Treatment

### Spleen vacuity pattern (*pi xu xing*)

**Disease causes:** Due to weakness of their spleen and stomach, the child has indigestion which causes it to experience abdominal pain.

**Main signs & symptoms:** Night crying every night occurring soon after birth and lasting for several months, curled, cold limbs, a pale, bluish facial complexion which is especially blue between the eyebrows and around the lips, poor appetite, and loose stools

**Treatment principles:** Strengthen the spleen, supplement the center, and promote digestion

**Treatment methods:**

1. Slightly bend the child's thumb and rub the line on the lateral palmar edge of the thumb, pushing in one direction only from the tip to the base of the thumb 100-500 times. (Fig. 221) This is called supplementing the Spleen Channel. Stimulation of this point in this manner strengthens the spleen and supplements the center, thus strengthening and promoting the digestion.

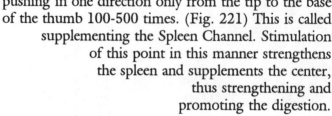

**Figure 221**

2. Knead the point in the center of the back of the hand 100-300 times. (Fig. 222) This is called kneading the Outer Palace of Labor. Stimulation of this point warms yang and disperses cold and especially warms the lower burner.

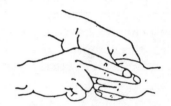

**Figure 222**

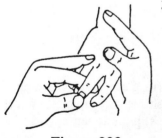

3. Knead the point at the middle of the crease on the back of the wrist 100-300 times. (Fig. 223) This is called kneading the Number One Nest of Wind. Stimulation of this point warms the middle burner, moves the qi, and relieves abdominal distention and pain.

**Figure 223**

4. Nip and knead the point at the center of the base of the palm where major and minor eminences (*i.e.*, bulges) meet. Nip 3-5 times and knead 50-100 times. (Fig. 224 below) This is called nipping and kneading the Small Heavenly Heart. Stimulation of this point calms the spirit, opens the portals, and eliminates stasis.

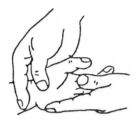

**Figure 224**

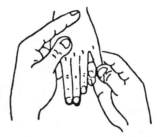

**Figure 225**

5. Nip with one's thumbnail and knead with the tip of the thumb the points on the middle knuckles of all five fingers on the back side of the hand. Nip 3-5 times and knead 30-500 times each. (Fig. 225) These points are called the *Wu Zhi Jie* (Five Finger Joints). This maneuver is, therefore, called nipping and kneading the Five Finger Joints. Stimulation of these points quiets the spirit and relieves convulsions.

6. Rub the line on the lateral anterior surface of the forearm, pushing in one direction only from the wrist to the elbow 100-300 times. (Fig. 226) This is called pushing the Three Gates. Stimulation of this point supplements the qi and fortifies yang.

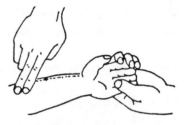

**Figure 226**

7. Round rub the abdomen around the navel counterclockwise with the hollow of the palm 100-500 times. (Fig. 227) This is called round rubbing the Abdomen. Stimulation of this point in this manner supplements the center and strengthens digestion.

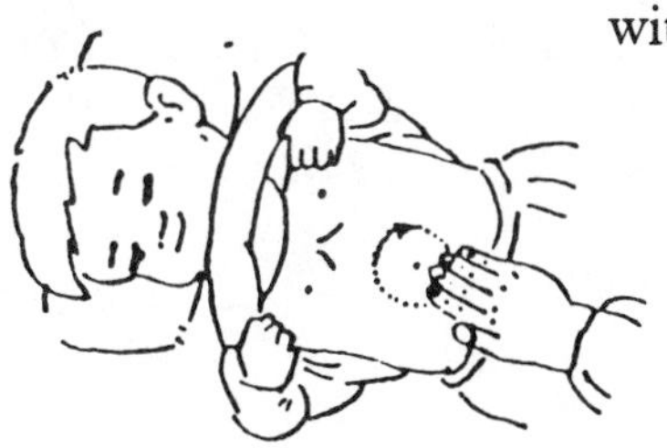

**Figure 227**

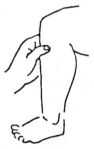

**Figure 228**

8. Knead the point below the knee on the lateral surface of the lower leg in between the tibia and fibula 50-100 times on both legs. (Fig. 228) This is called kneading Three *Li*. Stimulation of this point harmonizes the stomach and intestines and promotes digestion.

## Heat bind pattern (*re jie xing*)

**Disease causes:** The child's tendency to excessive yang qi combined with their inherent digestive immaturity and weakness

**Main signs & symptoms:** Crying every night which is loud and forceful, constipation, dark colored, difficult to void urination, restlessness, a flushed face and red lips

**Treatment principles:** Clear heat, quiet the spirit, and promote bowel movements

**Treatment methods:**

1. Rub the line on the tip of the palmar surface of the middle finger, pushing in one direction only from the transverse crease of the third knuckle to the tip 100-300 times. (Fig. 229) This point is called *Xin Jing* (Heart Channel) and this maneuver is called slightly draining the Heart Channel. Stimulation of this point clears heart fire and quiets the spirit.

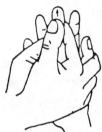

**Figure 229**

2. Rub the line on the medial (*i.e.*, ulnar), palmar edge of the little finger, pushing in one direction only from the base to the tips 100-300 times. (Fig. 230) This is called slightly draining the small intestine channel. Stimulation of this point in this manner clears heat from the heart by draining the small intestine with which it is connecting in an exterior/interior relationship.

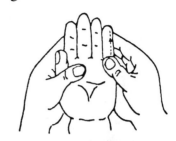

**Figure 230**

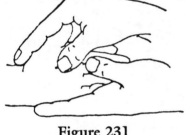

**Figure 231**

3. Knead the point at the center of the palm 100-300 times. (Fig. 231) This point is called *Nei Lao Gong* (Inner Palace of Labor). It is the same as acupuncture point Per 8. This maneuver is called kneading the Inner Palace of Labor. Stimulation of this point clears heat and relieves the exterior as well as relieves convulsions.

4. Nip and knead the point at the base of the palm where the major and minor eminences (*i.e.*, bulges) meet. Nip 3-5 times and knead 50-100 times. (Fig. 232) This is called nipping and kneading the Small Heavenly Heart. Stimulation of this point quiets the spirit.

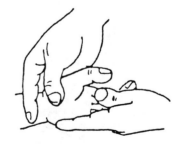

**Figure 232**

131

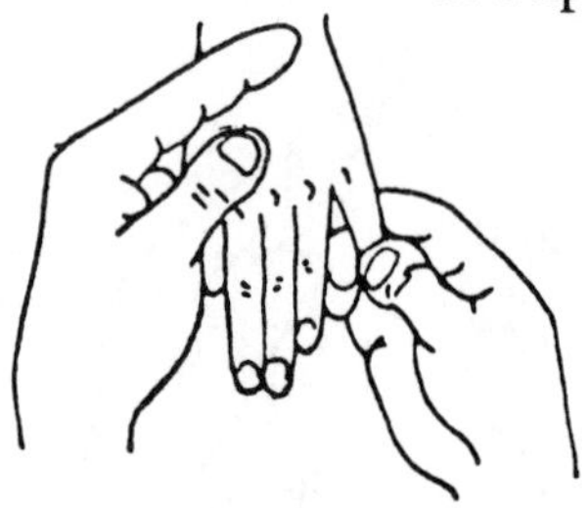

5. Nip with the thumbnail and knead with the thumb the points located on the middle knuckles on the backs of the five fingers. Nip 3-5 times and knead 30-50 times. (Fig. 233) this is called nipping and kneading the Five Finger Joints. Stimulation of these points quiets the spirit and relieves convulsions.

**Figure 233**

6. Knead the point in the center of the crease of the wrist on the palmar surface of the hand 100-300 times. (Fig. 234) This point is called *Zong Jin* (Ancestral Sinew). It is also called *Da Ling* (Great Mound). It is the same as acupuncture point Per 7. This maneuver is called kneading the Ancestral Sinew. Stimulation of this point clears heat, relieves spasms, and quiets the spirit.

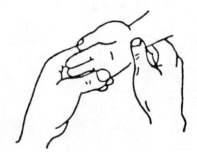

**Figure 234**

7. Rub the line on the midline of the anterior surface of the forearm, pushing in one direction only from the wrist to the elbow 100-300 times. (Fig. 235) This is called pushing the Milky Way. Stimulation of this point clears heat, relieves the exterior, and drains fire.

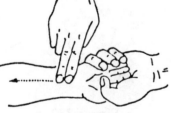

**Figure 235**

132

8. Round rub the abdomen around the navel clockwise with the hollow of the palm 100-500 times. (Fig. 236) This is called round rubbing the Abdomen. Stimulation of this point in this manner promotes digestion and bowel movements.

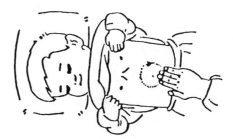

**Figure 236**

# Fright pattern (*jing xing*)

**Disease causes:** The inherent instability of the infant's spirit

**Main signs & symptoms:** Sudden crying with restlessness due to fright during sleep, timidness which can be relieved by being carried about in the arms, changeable face and lip color

**Treatment principles:** Clear heat, quiet the spirit, and relieve spasms and fright

**Treatment methods:**

1. Rub the line on the tip of the palmar surface of the index finger, pushing in one direction only from the transverse crease of the third knuckle to the tip 100-300 times. (Fig. 237) This point is called *Gan Jing* (Liver Channel) and this maneuver is called slightly draining the Liver Channel. Stimulation of this point in this manner clears heat from the liver and gallbladder, quiets the *hun* or ethereal soul, and relieves convulsions.

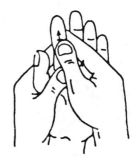

**Figure 237**

133

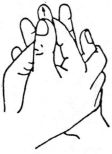

**Figure 238**

2. Rub the line on the tip of the palmar surface of the middle finger, pushing in one direction only from the transverse crease of the third knuckle to the tip 100-300 times. (Fig. 238) This is called slightly draining the Heart Channel. Stimulation of this point in this manner clears heat from the heart and quiets the spirit.

3. Rub the line on the tip of the palmar surface of the ring finger, pushing in one direction only from the transverse crease of the third knuckle to the tip 100-500 times. (Fig. 239) This is called slightly draining the Lung Channel. Stimulation of this point in this manner clears heat from the lungs.

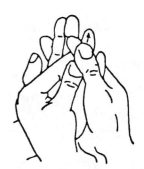

**Figure 239**

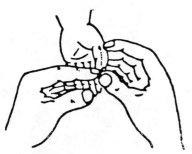

**Figure 240**

4. Slightly bend the child's thumb and rub the line on the lateral palmar edge of the thumb, pushing in one direction only from the tip of the thumb to its base, 100-500 times. (Fig. 240) This is called supplementing the Spleen Channel. Stimulation of this point in this manner supplements the spleen and harmonizes the stomach.

5. Nip and knead the point at the middle of the base of the palm where the major and minor eminences (*i.e.*, bulges) meet. Nip 3-5 times and knead 50-100 times. (Fig. 241) This is called nipping and kneading the Small Heavenly Heart. Stimulation of this point quiets the spirit, opens the portals, clears heat, stops convulsions, and eliminates stasis.

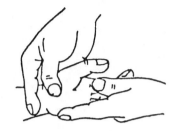

**Figure 241**

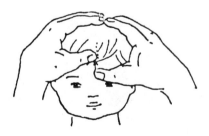

6. Nip with the thumbnail and knead with the thumb the points on the middle knuckles of the five fingers on the back of the hand. Nip 3-5 times and knead 30-50 times. (Fig. 242) This is called nipping and kneading the Five Finger Joints. Stimulation of these points quiets the spirit and relieves convulsions.

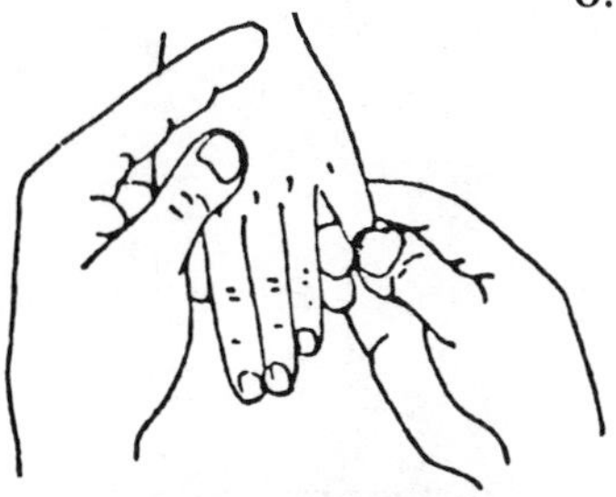

**Figure 242**

7. Gently rub the soft spot just above the forehead (*i.e.*, the anterior fontanelle) thumb over thumb from the front hairline backwards 50-100 times. (Fig. 243) If the fontanelle is not yet closed, only push to its forward edge. This point is called *Xin Men* (Heart Gate) and this maneuver is called pushing the Heart Gate. Stimulation of this point quiets the spirit.

**Figure 243**

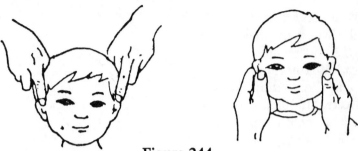

**Figure 244**

8. Grasp and lift the tips of both ears with index and middle fingers 30-50 times. Then grasp and pull downward both earlobes with thumbs and index fingers 30-50 times. (Fig. 244) This is called *Yuan Hou Zhai Guo* (Ape Picking Fruit). Stimulation of this point quiets the spirit.


# Food damage pattern (*shang shi xing*)

**Disease causes:** Overfeeding impairs digestion

**Main signs & symptoms:** Sudden night crying, abdominal distention, vomiting, and fetid smelling stools

**Treatment principles:** Harmonize the stomach and intestines, eliminate accumulations, and promote bowel movements

**Treatment methods:**

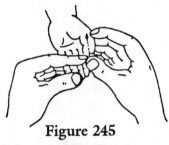

**Figure 245**

1. Slightly extend the child's thumb and rub the lateral palmar edge of the thumb, pushing in one direction only from the tip to the base 100-300 times. (Fig. 245) This is called supplementing the Spleen Channel. Stimulation of this point in this manner removes food stagnation and promotes digestion by strengthening the spleen.

2. Rub the line on the lateral palmar edge of the index finger, pushing in one direction only from the base to its tip 100-300 times. (Fig. 246) This is called slightly draining the Large Intestine Channel. Stimulation of this point in this manner clears heat from the intestines and frees the bowels.

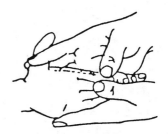

**Figure 246**

3. Knead the major bulge (*i.e.*, the thenar eminence) at the base of the thumb 100-300 times. (Fig. 247) This is called kneading the Shuttered Gate. Stimulation of this point in this manner removes food stagnation and promotes digestion.

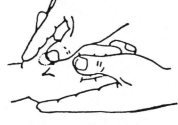

**Figure 247**

4. Rub the circle on the palm of the hand 100-300 times. This circle's center is the center of the palm and its radius is 2/3 the length from the center to the transverse crease at the base of the middle finger. (Fig. 248) This is called moving or transporting the Eight Trigrams. Stimulation of this point in this manner rectifies and frees the flow of qi and blood as well as harmonizes the functions of the five major organs.

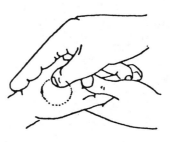

**Figure 248**

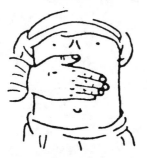

**Figure 249**

5. Knead the point above the navel with the hollow of the palm clockwise 100-300 times. (Fig. 249) This is called kneading the Central Venter. Stimulation of this point in this manner harmonizes the stomach and removes stagnation.

6. With both thumbs, obliquely push apart along the curves of the ribs from the upper abdomen to the sides of the belly 100-300 times. (Fig. 250) Stimulation of this point strengthens the spleen and stomach and promotes digestion.

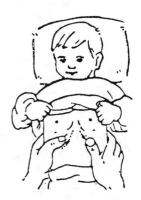

**Figure 250**

7. Knead the point below the knee on the lateral surface of the lower leg between the tibia and the fibula 50-100 times on both legs. (Fig. 251) This is called kneading Three *Li*. Stimulation of this point harmonizes the stomach and intestines and promotes digestion.

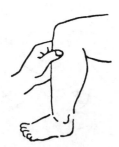

**Figure 251**

8. Rub the line on the center of the sacrum, pushing in one direction only from the small of the back to the tailbone 100-300 times. (Fig. 252) This is called pushing the Sacrum. Stimulation of this point in this manner promotes bowel movements.

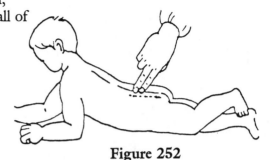

**Figure 252**

## Points for Special Attention

**1.** Parents should be made aware that sometimes night crying is due to simple conditions, such as hunger, thirst, a wet diaper, itching, being cold or hot, being stuck by a sharp object such as a diaper pin, chafing of the skin, etc. Some children are accustomed to seeing light. When there is no light, the child cries. In such cases, turning a light on will stop the crying.

**2.** Avoid feeding the child any raw or cold or spicy, hot foods. All foods should be easily digestible. Also, do not overfeed the child.

**3.** The child's room should be quiet and away from potentially frightening noises.

**4.** The above infant *tui na* protocols are performed once per day. Three treatments equal one course. Typically, most children recover after one course of treatment. If there is no effect, 1-2 more courses of treatment should be given.

# General Infant Massage for a Healthy Baby

Pediatric *tui na* for promoting general health refers to using certain Chinese infant massage manipulations on certain points with the intention of improving the child's general health and preventing the occurrence of disease. Chinese infant massage can improve the appetite, strengthen the constitution, prevent disease, and promote growth. The manipulations to achieve these effects can be done anytime. They are easy to do and are painless. Thus, they are readily accepted by children.

## Treatment Methods

1. Slightly bend the child's thumb and rub the line on the lateral palmar edge of the thumb, pushing in one direction only from the tip of the thumb to its base 100-500 times. (Fig. 253) This is called supplementing the Spleen Channel. Stimulation of this point in this manner strengthens the spleen and supplements the center, thus strengthening the source of production of the qi and blood of the entire body.

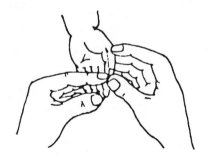

**Figure 253**

2. Round rub the abdomen around the navel counterclockwise 100-200 times and then clockwise 100-200 times. (Fig. 254 below) This is called round rubbing the

Abdomen. Stimulation of this point in this manner disperses accumulations and promotes bowel movements at the same time as it supplements the center and harmonizes the spleen and stomach.

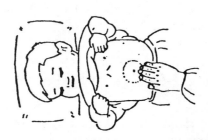

**Figure 254**

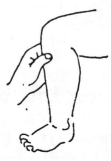

**Figure 255**

3. Knead the point below the knees on the lateral surface of the lower leg between the tibia and fibula 50-100 on both legs. (Fig. 255) This is called kneading Three *Li*. Stimulation of this point strengthens the spleen and supplements the center, harmonizes the spleen and stomach and promotes the digestion.

4. First apply some massage medium and lightly massage the center of the spine from above to below 3 times. Then place both hands on either side of the tailbone, grasping and lifting the skin with the thumbs and index and middle fingers, rolling the skin upward from the tailbone to the base of the neck in one direction only 3-5 times. (Fig. 256) This is called pinching and pulling the Spine. Stimulation of this point in this manner boosts the qi of the entire body and promotes the upbearing of clear yang.

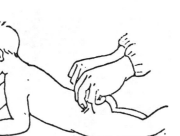

**Figure 256**

142

## Points for Special Attention

**1.** Generally, this infant massage protocol is appropriate to do once per day in the morning before breakfast. Seven such treatments equal one course of treatment. Another course can be done starting one day later. This protocol can help a constitutionally weak child or one prone to frequent illnesses to become stronger and more resistant to disease. It helps strengthen the digestion and improves the appetite at the same time as it eliminates food stagnation. Typically, a child's height and weight will increase after 3-6 months of therapy.

**2.** This massage protocol should be suspended whenever the child is suffering from an acute infectious disease. In such cases, the child should be treated with the appropriate remedial Chinese pediatric *tui na* regime. Once the illness has been cured, one can resume this protocol again.

# Concluding Words

Chinese infant massage or *xiao er tui na* has been practiced in China for hundreds of years. During those centuries, it has been used both to treat disease and to protect and promote infants' health. Chinese pediatric *tui na* is a simple yet effective skill that can be learned and practiced by parents and professional health care practitioners alike. It is a treasure benefitting the future of mankind — our children — and deserves to be passed from generation to generation and from people to people.

## Going Further

Hopefully this small book will help English-speaking parents and practitioners get started with Chinese infant massage. For more information on this art, the interested reader should see:

> *Infantile Tuina Therapy* by Luan Chang-ye, Foreign Languages Press, Beijing
> *Chinese Pediatric Practitioners Reference Manual*, and *A Parent's Guide to Chinese Pediatric Massage* (book and video), by Kyle Cline, Institute of Traditional Medicine, Portland Oregon
> *Chinese Bodywork: A Complete Handbook of Chinese Therapeutic Massage,* by Sun Cheng-nan, Pacific View Press, Berkeley, CA

For more information on Chinese pediatrics, please see:
> *Essentials of Traditional Chinese Pediatrics* by Cao Ji-ming *et al.*, Foreign Languages Press, Beijing
> *The English-Chinese Encyclopedia of Practical Traditional Chinese Medicine, Vol. 13, Pediatrics,* edited by Qi Xiu-heng, Higher Education Press, Beijing

For more information on Chinese medicine in general, the reader is referred to:
> *The Web That Has No Weaver* by Ted Kaptchuk, Congdon & Weed, NY

# Index

# OTHER BOOKS ON CHINESE MEDICINE
# AVAILABLE FROM BLUE POPPY PRESS
### 3450 Penrose Place, Suite 110, Boulder, CO  80301
### For ordering 1-800-487-9296  PH. 303\447-8372 FAX 303\245-8362

**A NEW AMERICAN ACUPUNCTURE** by Mark Seem, ISBN 0-936185-44-9

**ACUPOINT POCKET REFERENCE** ISBN 0-936185-93-7

**ACUPUNCTURE AND MOXIBUSTION FORMULAS & TREATMENTS** by Cheng Dan-an, trans. by Wu Ming, ISBN 0-936185-68-6

**ACUTE ABDOMINAL SYNDROMES: Their Diagnosis & Treatment by Combined Chinese-Western Medicine** by Alon Marcus, ISBN 0-936185-31-7

**AGING & BLOOD STASIS: A New Approach to TCM Geriatrics** by Yan De-xin, ISBN 0-936185-63-5

**AIDS & ITS TREATMENT ACCORDING TO TRADITIONAL CHINESE MEDICINE** by Huang Bing-shan, trans. by Fu-Di & Bob Flaws, ISBN 0-936185-28-7

**BETTER BREAST HEALTH NATURALLY with CHINESE MEDICINE** by Honora Lee Wolfe & Bob Flaws ISBN 0-936185-90-2

**THE BOOK OF JOOK: Chinese Medicinal Porridges, An Alternative to the Typical Western Break- fast** by B. Flaws, ISBN0-936185-60-0

**CHINESE MEDICAL PALMISTRY: Your Health in Your Hand** by Zong Xiao-fan & Gary Liscum, ISBN 0-936185-64-3

**CHINESE MEDICINAL TEAS: Simple, Proven, Folk Formulas for Common Diseases & Promoting Health** by Zong Xiao-fan & Gary Liscum, ISBN 0-936185-76-7

**CHINESE MEDICINAL WINES & ELIXIRS** by Bob Flaws, ISBN 0-936185-58-9

**CHINESE PEDIATRIC MASSAGE THERAPY**: *A Parent's & Practitioner's Guide to the Prevention & Treatment of Childhood Illness* by Fan Ya-li, ISBN 0-936185-54-6

**CHINESE SELF-MASSAGE THERAPY: The Easy Way to Health** by Fan Ya-li ISBN 0-936185-74-0

**A COMPENDIUM OF TCM PATTERNS & TREATMENTS** by Bob Flaws & Daniel Finney, ISBN 0-936185-70-8

**CURING ARTHRITIS NATURALLY WITH CHINESE MEDICINE** by Douglas Frank & Bob Flaws ISBN 0-936185-87-2

**CURING DEPRESSION NATURALLY WITH CHINESE MEDICINE** by Rosa Schnyer & Bob Flaws ISBN 0-936185-94-5

**CURING HAY FEVER NATURALLY WITH CHINESE MEDICINE** by Bob Flaws, ISBN 0-936185-91-0

**CURING HEADACHES NATURALLY WITH CHINESE MEDICINE**, by Bob Flaws, ISBN 0-936185-95-3

**CURING INSOMNIA NATURALLY WITH CHINESE MEDICINE** by Bob Flaws ISBN 0-936185-85-6

**CURING PMS NATURALLY WITH CHINESE MEDICINE** by Bob Flaws ISBN 0-936185-85-6

KEEPING YOUR CHILD HEALTHY
WITH CHINESE MEDICINE by Bob Flaws,
ISBN 0-936185-71-6

THE LAKESIDE MASTER'S STUDY OF
THE PULSE by Li Shi-zhen, trans. by Bob
Flaws, ISBN 1-891845-01-2

Li Dong-yuan's TREATISE ON THE
SPLEEN & STOMACH, A Translation of the
Pi Wei Lun by Yang Shou-zhong & Li Jian-yong, ISBN 0-936185-41-4

LOW BACK PAIN: Care & Prevention
with Chinese Medicine by Douglas Frank, ISBN 0-936185-66-X

MASTER HUA'S CLASSIC OF THE CEN-
TRAL VISCERA by Hua Tuo, ISBN 0-936185-43-0

MASTER TONG'S ACUPUNCTURE: An
Ancient Alternative Style in Modern Clinical Practice by
Miriam Lee 0-926185-37-6

THE MEDICAL I CHING: Oracle of the
Healer Within by Miki Shima, OMD, ISBN 0-936185-38-4

MANAGING MENOPAUSE NATU-
RALLY with Chinese Medicine by Honora
Lee Wolfe ISBN 0-936185-98-8

PAO ZHI: Introduction to Processing Chinese Medicinals to Enhance Their Therapeu-
tic Effect, by Philippe Sionneau, ISBN 0-936185-62-1

PATH OF PREGNANCY, VOL. I, Gesta-
tional Disorders by Bob Flaws, ISBN 0-936185-39-2

PATH OF PREGNANCY, Vol. II, Post-
partum Diseases by Bob Flaws. ISBN 0-936185-42-2

PEDIATRIC BRONCHITIS: Its Cause,
Diagnosis & Treatment According to TCM
trans. by Gao Yu-li and Bob Flaws, ISBN 0-936185-26-0

PRINCE WEN HUI'S COOK: Chinese Di-
etary Therapy by Bob Flaws & Honora Lee
Wolfe, ISBN 0-912111-05-4, $12.95 (Published by
Paradigm Press)

THE PULSE CLASSIC: A Translation of
the Mai Jing by Wang Shu-he, trans. by Yang
Shou-zhong ISBN 0-936185-75-9

THE SECRET OF CHINESE PULSE DI-
AGNOSIS by Bob Flaws, ISBN 0-936185-67-8

SEVENTY ESSENTIAL TCM FORMU-
LAS FOR BEGINNERS by Bob Flaws, ISBN 0-936185-59-7

SHAOLIN SECRET FORMULAS for
Treatment of External Injuries, by De Chan,
ISBN 0-936185-08-2

STATEMENTS OF FACT IN TRADI-
TIONAL CHINESE MEDICINE by Bob
Flaws, ISBN 0-936185-52-X

STICKING TO THE POINT 1: A Rational
Methodology for the Step by Step Formula-
tion & Administration of an Acupuncture
Treatment by Bob Flaws ISBN 0-936185-17-1

STICKING TO THE POINT 2: A Study of
Acupuncture & Moxibustion Formulas and
Strategies by Bob Flaws ISBN 0-936185-97-X

A STUDY OF DAOIST ACUPUNCTURE
by Liu Zheng-cai ISBN 1-891845-08-X

TEACH YOURSELF TO READ MODERN
MEDICAL CHINESE by Bob Flaws, ISBN 0-936185-99-6

THE SYSTEMATIC CLASSIC OF ACU-
PUNCTURE  & MOXIBUSTION (Jia Yi Jing)
by Huang-fu Mi, trans. by Yang Shou-zhong & Charles
Chace, ISBN 0-936185-29-5

THE TAO OF HEALTHY EATING
ACCORDING TO CHINESE MEDICINE by
Bob Flaws, ISBN 0-936185-92-9